THE BIG BOOK OF MEDICINE

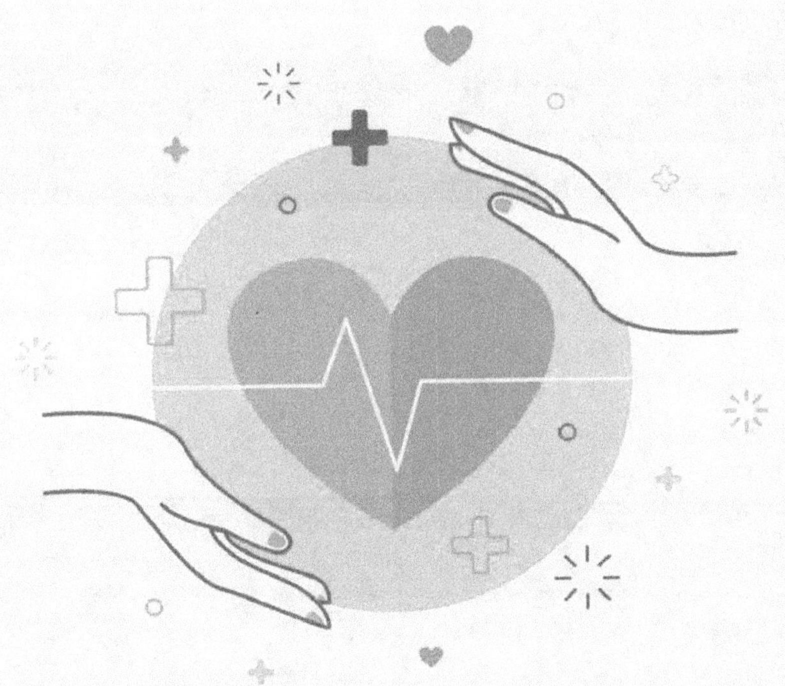

David Holman

Contents

Contents

Contents

Contents

Preventive dentistry

Scaling and cleaning

Drilling and filling

Dental trauma

Extractions

Prosthetics

Contents

What is Ketamine?

How do I debride a wound?

Can I give resuscitation fluids rectally?

How do I amputate a leg?

Can I use Superglue to close a wound?

How do I know if someone is dead?

Why is diarrhoea important?

How likely is an infectious disease like SARS or a new strain of influenza to cause a major disaster?

What is influenza? What is "Bird flu"? Will Tamiflu save me from the Pandemic? How do I use maggots to clean a wound? Can I use sugar to treat an infected wound? How do I "set" a broken bone?

How do I recognise and treat a heart attack in an austere situation? Do I need Quickclot or Traumadex to control bleeding?

What is the most useful antibiotic?

Contents

What do I do if I'm allergic to penicillin? When should I stop using antibiotics?

Background

This book is a major revision of the Survival Medicine FAQ's (Frequently Asked Questions) originally written for the misc. survivalism Usenet newsgroup in 1997. It was written in response to recurring posts asking the same questions and the fact that many answers were often wrong and occasionally dangerous. It hasn't undergone any changes or revisions since then.

Contents

While the original content remains valid we thought it was time it underwent an update. This is a significant revision – most sections have been re-written and a number of new sections added. We hope you will find it useful. It is offered in good faith but the content should be validated and confirmed from other sources before being relied on even in an emergency situation.

There are very few books aimed at the "Practicing Medicine after the End of the World As We Know It" market – which is hardly surprising! So we hope this book fills a void. We also hope it will be useful for those people delivering health care in remote or austere environments.

It is not designed as a "how to do x" reference – although there is some of that. There are plenty of books which tell you how to practice medicine. It is designed to provide some answers to commonly asked questions relating to survival/preparedness medicine and to provide relevant information not commonly found in traditional texts or direct you to that information.

We have tried to minimise technical language, but at times this has not been possible, if you come across unfamiliar terms – please consult a medical dictionary.

It has taken two years, and a lot of stopping, and starting but here it is. The authors and editors are passionately committed to helping people develop their medical knowledge and skills for major disasters. We hope you find it useful.

Web Site:

For questions and comments the authors can all be contacted via posting at the following website:

SurvivalistInc.com

Medicine at the End of the World

"With no antibiotics there would be no treatment for bacterial infections; pneumonia or a simple cut could kill again, contagious diseases (including those sexually transmitted) would make a come back, and high mortality rates would be associated with any surgery. Poor hygiene and disrupted water supplies would lead to an increase in diseases such as typhoid and cholera. Without vaccines there would be a progressive return in infectious diseases such as polio, tetanus, whooping cough, diphtheria, mumps, etc. especially among children. People suffering from chronic illnesses such as asthma, diabetes, or epilepsy would be severely affected with many dying (especially insulin-dependent diabetics). There would be no anaesthetic agents resulting in return to tortuous surgical procedures with the patient awake or if they were lucky drunk or stoned. The same would apply to painkillers; a broken leg would be agony, and dying of cancer would be distressing for the patient and their family.

Contents

Without reliable oral contraceptives or condoms the pregnancy rate would rise and with it the maternal and neonatal death rates, women would die during pregnancy and delivery again, and premature babies would die. Women would still seek abortions, and without proper instruments or antibiotics death from septic abortion would be common again. In the absence of proper dental care teeth would rot, and painful extractions would have to be performed. What limited medical supplies available would have to be recycled, resulting in increasing risks of hepatitis and HIV infection."

Chapter 1 Introduction

What is preparedness/survival medicine? Our definition is: "The practice of medicine in an environment or situation where standard medical care and facilities are unavailable, often by persons with no formal medical training". This includes medical care while trekking in third world countries, deep-water ocean sailing, isolated tramping and trekking, and following a large natural disaster or other catastrophe.

The basic assumption is that trained doctors and hospital care will be unavailable for a prolonged period of time, and that in addition to providing first aid - definitive medical care and rehabilitation (if required) will need to be provided. Also the basics of personal and public hygiene will also need to be considered.

Austere medicine is the provision of medical care without access to modern investigations or technology.

As is the case with any aspects of preparedness you need to decide what you are preparing for and plan accordingly. For some it will only be a 72-hour crisis, for others it will be a major long-term event, and for yet others a multiple generation scenario. Your medical preparations will need to reflect your own risk assessments in terms of what knowledge and skills you develop and what supplies/equipment/medicines you store. This book is more slanted towards preparation for medium to longer term disasters. But most of the included information is applicable to shorter situations as well.

A recent Internet survey asking about medical risk assessments in a major disaster came up with the following results:

"What do you see as the most likely common source of medical problems?

Contents

Battlefield injuries   5 %

Lack of surgical care   36 %

Environmental related   8 %

Infectious disease (naturally occurring)   64 %

Infectious disease (biological warfare)   20 %

Nuclear conflict (radiation, blast, burns)   4 % "

(Frugal's forum 1/04 with permission. http://www.frugalsquirrels.com)

What you may have to deal with will depend on what happens. Obviously a nuclear war will produce a di erent set of problems than a pandemic. However, regardless of whatever the initial triggering event after the initial wave of injuries or illness associated with it the majority of medical problems that happen will be common, and mundane, and not nearly as interesting as the above survey results suggests.

Below are the results of one author's experience in the provision of health care in various remote and austere locations (some third world, some first world) to nearly two thousand people over a cumulative 15-month period (spread over 10 years). The record keeping was a bit unreliable at times, but the following summary is reasonably accurate.

The Top 20 presentations:

Contents

Top 12 prescribed drugs:

The above gives you a variety of insights into what medical problems might occur and what medications are likely to be required. Most of it relatively mundane and not life threatening. Truly catastrophic problems in medicine are fortunately rare. You should focus on dealing with the common problems, and doing common procedures well, and you will save lives, and improve the quality of people's lives. While major trauma and surgical emergencies occur – they are reassuringly not that common. To deal with these will require additional knowledge and resources over and above what is require to safely manage 95% of common medical problems.

Perhaps the single most important piece of advice in this book:

While the focus of this book is on practicing medicine in an austere environment it does not address one key area which must be considered as part of your preparations: That is optimising your health prior to any disaster; losing weight, keeping fit, maintaining a healthy diet, and managing any chronic health problem aggressively.

This is well covered in 100s of books about getting fit and staying healthy, but if you do not take some action in this regard all of your other preparations may be in vain when you drop dead of a heart attack from the stress of it all.

Chapter 2: What do I need to know and how do I learn it?

The more you learn the better! Start off learning basic first aid. Then try and learn as much anatomy and physiology as possible –A & P are the building blocks of medicine. Once you understand how the body is put together and how it works you are in a much better position to understand disease and injury and apply appropriate treatments. Then you should try and obtain some more advanced medical education and practical experience.

There is no syllabus that we can list that will tell you what you need to know to cover every eventuality. Table 2.1 contains some core basic knowledge skills, which should be considered fundamental to anyone assuming responsibility for providing medical care.

While having a list of core knowledge is helpful. Ultimately what you need to be able to do is: "Know how to perform a basic assessment, established a rough working diagnosis, and know where to look to find further information about what to do next." The fact you don't know all the fine print doesn't matter, the key is having a rough idea of what is going on, and knowing where to look to find out more, and ensuring you have the references available.

Medicine is dangerous, and uninformed decisions and actions will kill people. Despite having said that a lot of medicine is simply common sense. Anyone with a bit of intelligence, a good A&P book, and a good basic medical text can easily learn the basics. The ideal is a trained health care professional and anything else is taking risks, but in a survival situation any informed medical care is better than no medical care.

Please note we say informed; if you really don't have a clue what you are doing you will be very dangerous.

Formal training

Professional medical training: The ideal option is undertaking college study in a medical area e.g. Medicine, Nursing, Physicians Assistant, Paramedic, Vet, etc. This clearly isn't an option for many, but it is still the best option and should be clearly identified as such.

Other Formal training options by region:

N.B In the following sections a number of commercial courses are mentioned. We have no financial interest in any of these courses. While we have heard positive things about the commercial courses mentioned we do not offer any endorsement of any

Table 2.1 Core knowledge and skills to aim for

Contents

- - Use a good medical dictionary and a basic medical textbook to answer questions – know where to look to find answers to things you don't know.
  - Perform basic bandaging and dressings. Clean a wound, debride a burn.
  - Use local anaesthetic to numb a wound.
  - Debride and suture a wound, but also know when not to suture a wound, and leave it open or perform delayed closure.
  - Deliver a baby and afterbirth. Suture a vaginal tear, manage a post-partum bleed.
  - Reduce and immobilise a short and long bone fracture/dislocation.
  - Use basic counselling skills.
  - Understand basic hygiene and preventive medicine practices.
  - Recognise and treat common infections:
    - Viral flu
    - Upper respiratory tract infections
    - Pneumonia
    - Urinary infection
    - Wound or skin infection
    - Common STD's
  - Recognise and treat common medical and surgical problems:
    - Asthma/respiratory distress
    - Abdominal pain – renal (kidney) stones/appendix/biliary stones
    - Allergic reactions/anaphylaxis
  - Look after some one who is bed bound, e.g. basic nursing care, managing the unconscious patient, catheterisation.
  - Use basic dental skills, simple fillings, infections, and extractions.
  - Insert an IV and understand basic fluid resuscitation.
  - Improvise medical equipment and supplies.

Contents

particular course or any warrantee as to the quality of the teaching provided. Times change and good things can and do go bad. When looking at a particular course look in detail at what is being covered (e.g. is it a national standard? Does it cover what you need to know?) And who are the instructors? (Do they have credibility? What are their backgrounds?)

United States:

EMT Basic: This is the national standard for providing Emergency care in the USA. The courses follow a curriculum set out by the US Dept of Transportation. They are offered by many community colleges. While in theory the content is the same, there is wide variation in quality of teaching over different sites. The best feedback you are likely to get will come from previous students. The course length is usually several hundred hours.

This is probably the minimum standard to aim for – it provides an overview of anatomy and physiology, and an introduction to the basics of looking after sick and injured patients. It is based around delivering the patient to a hospital as an end result so is of limited value in remote and austere medicine – but it provides a solid

introduction.

Additionally, the US recognizes various levels of EMT which we will generically call Intermediate and Paramedic;

EMT-Intermediates are generally allowed to initiate venous access and to administer a modest array of emergency drugs, use oesophageal and blind intubation airway devices such as the Combitube, and use automated defibrillators. Patient assessment skills are also more developed than with the EMT-B or First Responder. Overall training is approximately 400 hours in addition to the pre-requisite EMT-Basic course.

EMT-Paramedics constitute the highest level of training for most states. In addition to all previous skills accorded EMT-Bs and Is they may make use of a significantly larger array of medications including gaseous analgesia, paralytics and amnesics.

They may also perform airway intubation via direct visualization, perform 12-lead interpretive EKGs, and in some jurisdictions are trained as community health providers able to perform immunizations, reduce minor dislocations, and perform simple wound closure.

First Responder: If you are unable to undertake an EMT-B course, this provides the "lite" version. Covering similar material in much less detail it is a good start but not overly in-depth. The usual course length is 40-80 hours – most quality schools offer a 60+ hour course. Various community education groups offer the course and the Red Cross also offers a variation.

The next level down from first responder is a standard "First Aid" course offered by the Red Cross and many other organisations

Contents

EMT/Wilderness EMT Course: For most this is a much more realistic option than formal college training. These courses give a basic background in anatomy and physiology, medical terminology, and the essentials of emergency medicine. It provides the basis for additional self-directed learning. Most community colleges offer these courses. The basics are well covered in the "first responder"/First Aid courses, which although very elementary provide a good stepping stone to the more advanced courses while not requiring the same time commitments as a full EMT courses.

Tactical EMS: There are a number of courses available which focus on tactical EMS

– the provision of emergency care in hostile environment and for prolonged periods. Frequently they have a prerequisite of at least EMT-B and usually some practical experience in a tactical environment. However some provide more entry-level courses. The focus of these courses is primarily on trauma and combat associated injuries. The quality of these courses varies enormously.

The original tactical EMT programme was developed by the US Protective Services, Counter Narcotics, and Terrorism program (CONTOM). They offer both basic and advanced EMT-Tactical programmes. Typically they are accessed through law enforcement programmes.

Another highly recommended course is the Operational and Emergency Medical Skills course. (http://www.oems.org/index.html). This course is unfortunately only available to medical staff attached to the Department of Defence and other federal agencies. FEMA staff and those involved in their Emergency Response teams have attended.

Some other providers of these types of courses include: Insight training http://www.insightstraining.com

HK Tactical Medical Training http://www.tacticalmedicine.com/

Global Medical rescue Services: GMRS offer a variety of excellent courses in remote and tactical medicine. Occasional courses focused on preparedness type medicine are also offered. These courses are unique in catering specifically for survival situations and are highly endorsed. http://www.gmrsltd.com/

(Editors note: Potential conflict of interest. One of the Editors is involved at an instructor level and others have taken courses with GMRS Ltd.)

Canada

St. John Ambulance: SJA provides the bulk of private first response and basic EMT training in Canada. There are probably a number of other more advanced courses available but we have had difficulty obtaining information on them.

United Kingdom:

Contents

First aid certificate: Basic first aid course. This is usually 8-24 hours worth of instruction. This an excellent place to start for those with minimal experience. It is offered through St. John Ambulance, or the Red Cross, and a number of commercial providers. If you are a member of either organisation they provide much more comprehensive training up to EMT basic level.

BASICS: The British Association for Immediate Care Schemes runs several courses with provide extensions from basic first aid. While not specifically focused on preparedness medicine, they provide an opportunity for non-professionals to obtain teaching up to an EMT-P theory level – although lack the practical hours. They offer the basic Immediate Care course and the more advanced Pre-hospital Emergency Care course. Both are expensive. They are also affiliated with the Faculty of Pre-Hospital of the Royal College of Surgeons of Edinburgh.

Basic surgical skills for remote medics: An intensive three-day course aimed at teaching the basics of surgical practise and to challenge the students with different problems using their newfound skills. Run by Remote Support Medics (http://www.remotemedics.co.uk) in association with The Royal College of Surgeons of Edinburgh.

Diploma in Remote and Offshore Medicine: Currently in development. Should be available in 2005. Aimed at medics working in the oil/gas industry at remote sites. This will become the gold standard for non-professional people in the UK getting experience for remote or austere medical work. (http://www.remotemedics.co.uk)

EMT / Advanced EMT: A number of different courses offered by Advanced Life Support Europe (http://www.advanced-lifesupport.com/). Their main gem is a 5-day clinical course in a UK hospital learning airway and IV skills which is available to non-professionals provided you have completed one of there pre-requisite courses. Their courses are unfortunately fairly expensive, but potentially very useful.

Expedition Medicine: This is one of several courses available in the UK focused on providing care in remote environments. It appears to be the only course available to non-doctors and nurses. (http://www.voyageconcepts.co.uk/expemed.htm)

Australia / New Zealand:

First aid certificate: Similar situation to the UK. Run by St. John, Red Cross, and some private providers.

Wilderness first responder: This a 10-day course offered by the Wilderness Medicine Institute at various sites around Australia. Not delivered at a particularly advanced level, but goes well beyond a standard first aid course and is focused on remote work. (http://www.wmi.net.au)

Informal Training

Emergency Department Observing: It is possible to gain some experience observing or working in an ER. Many Emergency Departments regularly have a variety of people coming through for practical experience from army medics, to off-shore, island, forest service staff, to fishing boat medics. If you can provide a good reason for wanting to gain skills in the emergency room such as "sailing your boat to the South Pacific," then the potential to gain practical experience in suturing, inserting IV's, and burn management is there. In North America this is more difficult to arrange due to insurance issues. However, if you are not actually going to touch a patient and are just going to be there to observe then if you ask the right people it should be easy to arrange. While not the same as "hands on" experience, simply experiencing the sights and sounds of illness and injury will help prepare you for if you have to do it yourself.

Arrange some teaching: Another option is befriending (or recruiting) a health care professional and arranging classes through them. It is common for doctors to be asked to talk to various groups on different topics so an invitation to talk to a "tramping club" about pain relief or treating a fracture in the bush would not be seen as unusual.

Volunteering: Many ambulances and fire services have volunteer sections or are completely run by volunteers. Through these services you may be able to obtain formal EMT training and at the same time gain valuable practical skills and experience, overcome fear of dealing with acutely sick people and also work with some great people. Organisations such as the Red Cross, Search and Rescue units, or Ski patrols also offer basic first aid training, as well as training in disaster relief and outdoor skills. It is also often possible to arrange "ride alongs" with ambulance and paramedic units as the 3rd person on the crew and observe patient care even if you are not able to be involved.

Chapter 3 Organisational issues

If you are alone or just a couple then organising your medical care is relatively straightforward. However, the larger the group the more formalised and structured your medical care should be. Someone within the group ideally with a medical background should be appointed medic. Their role is to build up their skill and knowledge base to be able to provide medical care to the group. There should also be a certain amount of cross training to ensure that if the medic is the sick or injured one there is someone else with some advanced knowledge. The medic should also be responsible for the development and rotation of the medical stores, and for issues relating to sanitation and hygiene. In regard to medical matters and hygiene their decisions should be absolute, and their advice should only be ignored in the face of a strong tactical imperative.

How you deliver care will depend on the size of the group you are looking after. Small groups don't require a formal "sick-call" or clinic time; you provide care if and when required and fit it in around other jobs. For a larger group dedicated time is required for running clinics and other related medical tasks e.g. public health work and it may be a full time activity.

Risk Assessment/Needs Assessment:

As alluded to in the introduction what you plan for depends on what you are worried about. As part of your medical preparations you should undertake a detailed needs assessment. You should ask and answer the following questions (at least):

Contents

1. What am I preparing for?

Natural disasters; Nuclear war; Ice ages; Economic collapse; Peak oil, etc.

1. How many people will I be looking after?
2. What age range will I be looking after?
3. How long will we need to be independent for?
4. What are their pre-existing health problems?
5. What physical condition are they in?
6. What physical environment will I be living in?

Hot/Cold; Wet/Dry; Underground shelter/above ground, etc.

1. What level of medical care can I provide?
2. What additional training do I need? How do I get it?
3. What supplies do I need? How much of each?
4. Do I have sufficient reference books?
5. Have I considered how I will deal with difficult issues relating to practicing medicine: Confidentiality, death and dying, sexuality, scarcity of resources, etc.

Documentation:

Even in a survival situation documentation is important. You should keep a record of every patient you treat. What they complained of, the history and examination, what you diagnosed, and how you managed them, a very clear note of any drugs you administer, and a description of any surgical procedure you perform should all be recorded. Anyone with an ongoing problem should have a chronological record of their condition and treatment over time recorded. There are two reasons for this. First is that for the ongoing care of the patient often it is only possible to make a diagnosis by looking over a course of events within retrospect and it is also important to have a record of objective findings to compare to recognise any changes over time in the patient condition. Second is for legal reasons. If and when things return to normal it may be important to justify why certain decisions were made. Detailed notes from the time will make this easier. It is also useful to have medical records on members of your group prior to any event including things such as blood groups and any existing or potential medical problems.

One useful method of recording medical information is the S.O.A.P format. It can be used to document every patient encounter. It provides a structure which is easy to follow and understand

S. Subjective

What the patient has complained about and the history associated with it, e.g. A Headache for 2 days with associated fever, nausea, and a stiff neck.

Contents

O. Objective

What you find on examining the patient or from your investigations, e.g. A fever of 39 degrees, looks dehydrated and has a purple rash.

A. Assessment

This is your assessment of what is wrong with the patient after your history taking, examination, and investigations, e.g. Probably bacterial meningitis

P. Plan

Your management plan for the patient, e.g. IV antibiotics and fluids. Isolate from others.

It is easy to follow and provides a consistent format for documentation.

Physical Location:

Where possible you should have a dedicated clinic area. For both functional and infection control reasons it is worth having a dedicated area.

Key features where possible (and this is a wish list): Clean – and easy to keep clean

Adequate lighting – both generally and more focused for examinations

Adequate space and storage

Adequate work surfaces and an examination table or bed Privacy

Access to water – preferably hot Warm/Dry

Protection from threats – ballistic and environmental

Rationing and Scarcity:

Contents

The persisting survival theme of how you deal with the "have nots" when they approach you applies to medicine as much as to food and other supplies. Obviously complete isolation is one option but this is unlikely to be common. How do you deal with the stranger dumped on you with the gunshot wound or pneumonia? It's one thing to give them a meal, but do you give them the last of your IV antibiotics or your one dose of IV anaesthetic? You need to have thought about these things in advance. People can often "live off the land," and forage for food but they cannot forage for penicillin. It's also worth realising that these people may be more likely to be in poor general health and also carriers of infectious diseases. This raises the question of isolation vs. community involvement again. One possible option may be to quarantine the refugees for a period of time before any contact with your group. There is no perfect quarantine time frame – but 14 days should cover the vast majority of infectious diseases.

The doctor-patient relationship:

Another important area is that of confidentiality and trust. This is a cornerstone of any medical relationship. It may seem an odd thing to mention in regards to a preparedness situation but as all doctors, nurses and paramedics will tell you without trust you can't practice. You need to trust that what you tell your medic will go no further, and personal problems won't become dinnertime conversations. Obviously this has to be weighed against the "common good" of the group but unless it would place the group in danger there should be an absolute rule and practice of confidentiality.

Chapter 4 Medical Kits

What you stock up on should be related to what you know how to use and what you can obtain. There are potentially thousands of drugs, and different pieces of medical equipment, and you can't stock everything. Fortunately it is possible to manage 90% of medical problems with only a moderate amount of basic equipment and drugs.

Obviously the treatment may not be as high quality as that provided by a proper hospital but it may be life saving and reduce long term problems. For example; a general anaesthetic, an operation for an internal tibial nail, followed by pain management, and physiotherapy usually manages a broken tibia in a hospital setting. In a remote austere situation it can be managed by manipulation with analgesia, and immobilization with an external splint for 6-8 weeks, and as a result the patient may be in pain for a few weeks, and have a limp for life but still have a functioning leg. Also appendicitis has been treated with high-dose antibiotics when surgery has been unavailable such as on a submarine or in the Antarctic. Removal of an appendix has been done successfully many times under local anaesthesia. Although in each case management maybe sub-optimal and may have some risk in a survival situation it can be done and may be successful with limited medication and equipment.

Obtaining medical supplies:

Medications:

Obtaining medications can be difficult. The problem is two-fold. First is access and second is cost. Below are some suggestions for legally obtaining medicines for use in a survival medicine situation.

Contents

1. Talk to your doctor. Be honest explain exactly why and what you want, that you want to be prepared for any disaster and have some important basic meds available, for if medical care isn't freely available. Demonstrate an understanding of what each drug is for and that you know how to safely use it. This approach depends on your relationship with your doctor, and how comfortably you are discussing these issues. Although, I would suggest that you don't request narcotics the first time. Then return the meds when they have expired, this will confirm that you are not using them inappropriately.

2. Discuss with your MD your plans for a trekking holiday. Most MDs recognise the importance of an adequate medical kit if you are travelling in the 3rd world or doing isolated backpacking. Most would prescribe antibiotics, rehydration fluid, simple pain killers, anti-diarrhoea meds, antibiotic and fungal creams, and if climbing steroids, acetazolamide and furosemide for AMS (although these last 2 have limited roles in a survival situation). It is also worth requesting Malaria prophylaxis – the CDC recommends doxycycline for most regions.

3. Buy a boat. Australia, New Zealand, and the UK, require all boats sailing beyond coastal limits to carry a comprehensive medical kit. This includes antibiotics, strong narcotic analgesias, and a variety of other meds. Although not a legal requirement in the US, I imagine most MD's would happily equip an ocean going yacht with a comprehensive medical kit, especially if you can demonstrate a basic medical knowledge. The US Public Health service offers suggested medications and equipment, depending on numbers and expected isolation.

4. Prescription medicines are available over the counter in many third world countries. While purchasing them certainly isn't illegal, importation into your own country may well be. While it is unlikely that a single course of antibiotics would be a problem, extreme care should be exercised with more uncommon drugs or large amounts. Narcotics shouldn't be imported under any circumstances. Should you purchase drugs in the third (or second) world you need to be absolutely sure you are getting what you believe you are, the best way is to ensure that the medications are still sealed in the original manufactures packaging.

5. "Not for human consumption": Veterinary meds are widely available and are relatively cheap – you can by human grade antibiotics from many fish supply stores. Several books discuss obtaining them (Survivalist Medicine Chest. Ragnar Benson. Paladin Press is one), so I won't cover it in detail here. We cannot recommend this method, but obviously for some it is the only viable option. Generally speaking most veterinary drugs come from the same batches and factories as the human version, the only difference being in the labelling. This is the case for most common single-component drugs such as antibiotics. If you are going to purchase veterinary medications I strongly suggest only purchasing antibiotics or topical preparations and with the following cautions: (1) Make sure you know exactly what drug you are buying, (2) avoid preparations which contain combinations of drugs and also obscure drugs for which you can find no identical human preparation and (3) avoid drug preparations for specific animal conditions for which there is no human equivalent. Buy drugs which are generically identical to their human counterparts, e.g. Amoxicillin 500mg (Vet) = Amoxicillin 500mg (Human), etc. You use these at your own risk.

A recent discussion with a number of doctors suggests that options ii and iii would be acceptable to the majority of those spoken too. In fact many were surprisingly broad in what they would be prepared to supply in those situations. However, be warned the majority of the same group considered the preparedness/survivalism philosophy to be unhealthy!

Other medical supplies:

Obtaining general medical supplies is often easier. Basic bandages, and stethoscopes, etc. can be bought from any medical supply house. In the USA there is no federal law prohibiting the purchase of things like sutures, syringes, needles, IVs, etc. but some

states can make it difficult. In most other countries they are freely available. Try looking in the yellow pages for medical, or emergency medical supply houses, or veterinary supplies. A number of commercial survival outfitters offer first aid and medical supplies, however, I would shop around before purchasing from these companies as their prices, in my experience, are higher than standard medical suppliers. The above approaches for obtaining medicines can also be used for obtaining medical equipment if you do have problems. The most important point is to be able to demonstrate an understanding of how to use what you are requesting.

Pre-packaged Kits: Generally speaking it is considerably cheaper to purchase your own supplies and put together your own kit. The commercial kits cost 2-3 times more than the same kit would cost to put together yourself and frequently contain items which are of limited value. The more you buy the cheaper things become – consider buying in bulk.

Storage and Rotation of Medications

Medications can be one of the more expensive items in your storage inventory, and there can be a reluctance to rotate them due to this cost issue, and also due to difficulties in obtaining new stock.

Unfortunately drugs do have limited shelf life. It is a requirement for medications sold in the US (and most other first world countries) to display an expiration date. It is our experience that these are usually very easy to follow, without the confusing codes sometimes found on food products, e.g. -- Exp. 12/00=Expires December 2000.

We cannot endorse using medications which have expired, but having said that, the majority of medications are safe for at least 12 months following their expiration date. As with food the main problem with expired medicines is not that they become dangerous but that they lose potency over time and the manufacturer will no longer guarantee the dose/response effects of the drug. We discuss using expired medications in more detail in Chapter 11.

The important exception to this rule was always said to be the tetracycline group of antibiotics which could become toxic with time. However, it is thought that the toxicity with degrading tetracycline was due to citric acid which was part of the tablet composition. Citric acid is no longer used in the production of tetracycline, therefore, the dangers of toxicity with degradation of tetracycline is no longer a problem.

Aspirin and Epinephrine do break down over time to toxic metabolites and extreme care should be taken using these medications beyond their expiry dates.

Despite the above comments "Let the buyer beware." The expiry dates ARE there for a reason, and there are almost certainly other medications which do break down, and become toxic after their expiry date.

Contents

In addition, we recommend that if you are acquiring medications on a doctor's prescription that when you have the prescription filled you explain the medications are for storage (you don't need to say exactly what for), and request recently manufactured stock with distant expiration dates.

The ideal storage conditions for most medications are in a cool, dark, dry environment. These conditions will optimise the shelf life of the drugs. A small number of drugs require refrigeration to avoid loss of potency. These include insulin, ergometrine, oxytocin, and some muscle relaxants. Others such as diazepam rapidly lose potency if exposed to the light.

How much?

This is a very individual question. It depends upon what you are preparing for and the number of people you will be looking after. It is impossible to say how much is enough. In order get a rough idea of what you should stock – think of your worse case scenario and at least double or triple the amounts you calculate. Items which never go as far as you think they will include – gauze, tape, antibiotics, and sutures. If you have ever been hospitalised or had a close relative in hospital for even a relatively minor problem take a look at the billing account for medical supplies and drugs to get an idea how much can be consumed with even a relatively small problem. It is simple mathematics; drugs which you need to take more than once or twice a day disappear extremely fast – penicillin 4 times a day for 10 days on a couple of occasions quickly erodes your "large stock" of 100 tablets! The same number of ciprofloxacin required only twice a day last longer. Dosing frequency is worth considering when deciding amounts.

Specific Medical Kits

Everyone has an idea of what his or her perfect kit is and what he or she thinks is vital

- so there is no perfect kit-packing list. What is perfect for one person's situation and knowledge may not be perfect for yours. You need to build a kit that you are able to understand and use.

In this section we have looked at a basic first aid kit, a more broad-spectrum basic medical kit, and an advanced medical kit able to cope with most medical problems. These are not the perfect kits or the ideal packing list – but they give you some idea of what we consider are needed to provide varying levels of care.

There is also frequent confusion over which surgical instruments to buy, how many of each, and what some actually do so we have gone into more detail looking at some possible surgical and dental kits, and what level of care can be delivered with each.

Note:

Contents

1. We've tried to use the international generic names for drugs. However, there are some differences between the British and the US pharmacopoeias and where possible we have tried to include both e.g. Lignocaine (UK & Oz/NZ) = Lidocaine (US)
2. We have not included any quantities. This is dependent on what you are planning for and what you can afford. Unfortunately most medications require rotation with 1- 5 year shelf lives, making this a costly exercise, as they are not like food you can

rotate into the kitchen

1. Always store a supply of any medicines you take regularly. These do not feature on the packing-lists. However, it is vital to remember the blood pressure pills, thyroid hormones, allergy pills, contraceptive pills, asthma inhalers, or what ever you take regularly. Most doctors will issue additional prescriptions for regular medication to allow an extra supply at a holiday home or to leave a supply at work. The main problem likely to arise is covering the cost of the extra medication which may be expensive and not covered by insurance. If you have previously had severe allergic reactions consider having a supply of Epi-pens

Contents

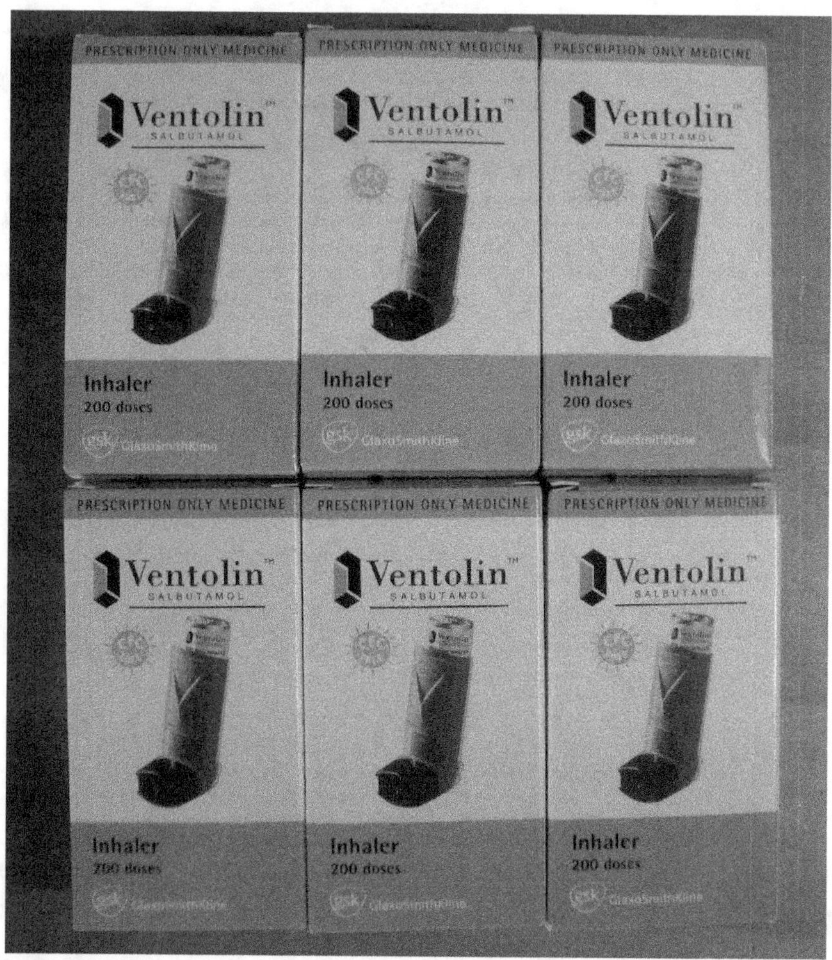

Figure 4.1. If you have a chronic medical problem such as asthma, you must ensure you have an adequate supply of your medication.

Contents

Before addressing what you need, it's worth looking at what you're going to put it in. There is large selection of medical bags on the market – military and civilian styles, rigid and soft construction. They vary in size from bum bags to large multi compartment backpacks and vary in price from less than $100 to more than $500 USD. We have selected 3-4 bags in each size range – personal use, first responder, and large multi-compartment bags. They cover a range of prices. What is right for you will depend on your individual requirements. If in a fixed location consider buying a rolling mechanics tool chest and using it as a "crash cart".

Personal size:

- o Battle pack (Chinook Medical gear)
  - o Modular Medical Pouch (Tactical Tailor)
  - o Compact individual medical pouch (S.O Tech) First responder size
  - o First response bag (Tactical Tailor)
  - o Modular bag system (Galls)
  - o Plano 747M Hard Case (Plano)
  - o NSW Medical Patrol bag (London Bridge Trading Company)
  - o Responder II (Conterra)
  - o Pelican waterproof case Large kit bag:
  - o M5 style bag (Tactical tailor)
  - o MIII Medical pack (Eagle)
  - o NSW Training/Coverage Medical Backpack (London Bridge Trading Company) - one of the best large bags on the market. The STOMP II Medical Backpack from Blackhawk industries is very similar to the NSW training/coverage pack from LBTC – but significantly cheaper.
  - o ALS pack (Conterra)
  - o Kifaru back-packs (Kifaru) – not specifically medical, but can be customised inside and out.

When you have selected the bags that suit you, one approach to organising your medical supplies is:

Contents

Personal bag: Carry this with you at all time. It contains basic first aid gear or in a tactical situation the equipment to deal with injuries from a gunshot wound or explosion. (figure 4.2)

First response bag: Carry this in your car; take it with you when you go camping etc. It contains more advanced first aid gear and some medical items.

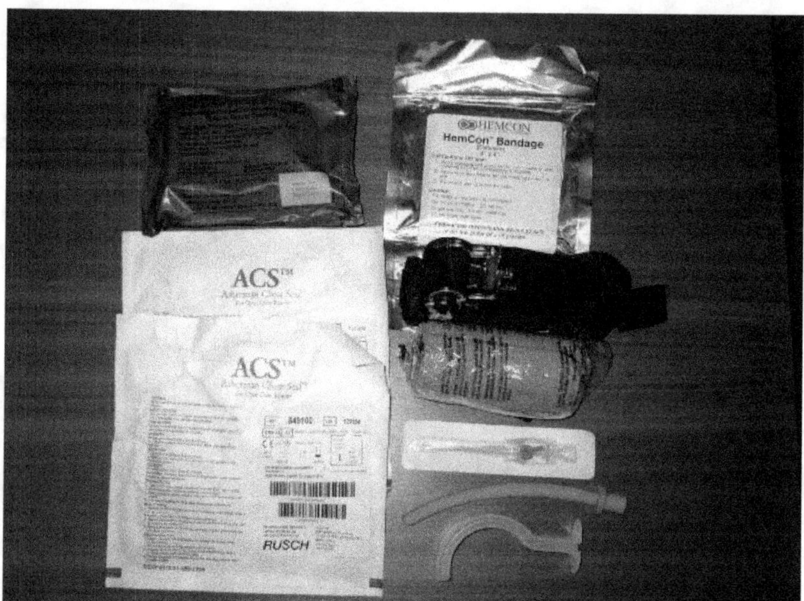

Figure 4.2 Blowout bag: Personal medical equipment for a tactical situation (Dressings, HemCon bandages, Asherman Chest seals, oral and nasal airways, iv cannular and a tourniquet).

Large kit bag: This is your home/retreat/bugging out medical kit. It contains your medical equipment as opposed to simple first aid supplies.

Storage area: In your home/retreat. It contains duplicate and bulk supplies. Large plastic storage bins are ideal for this.

Pack/organise/store items that are fragile, easily damaged by water, or can become messy (most liquids and ointments, ESPECIALLY tincture of benzoin in any form) in individual zip-lock plastic bags. For high-value water sensitive items (pulse oximeters, blood glucose meters, etc.) consider packing in water proof hard cases – such as the Pelican or Otter boxes.

Consider packing items that are used together into "battle-packs", ready to use packages – for example, pack an IV giving set with an IV start set with an Angio-Cath in zip-lock bag – so you can grab one thing and be ready to go.

Appendix 1 lists some medical suppliers.

EBay is a good source of medical supplies and surgical instruments but be careful to know what you are buying: Make certain you know what you want and what it would have cost from a supplier.

A brief note about airway management equipment

Before describing in detail packing lists for several possible kits we should discuss briefly airway management and the equipment associated with it. The details of this are best learnt in a First Aid /EMT class. The management of an airway has a number of steps:

- o Basic airway manoeuvres – head tilt, chin lift, jaw thrust.
  - o Simple airway adjuvants – oral airways, nasal airways.
  - o Advanced airway adjuvants – laryngeal masks, Combitubes.
  - o Endotracheal intubation – this is the gold standard of airway management. A plastic tube from the mouth into the trachea through which a patient can be ventilated.

In addition once you have managed the airway you need to ventilate the patient either with mouth-to-mouth/mask or using a mask - self inflating bag combination (e.g.

Ambubag).

The reason for discussing this is that you need to decide how much airway equipment to stock. Our view is that there is relatively little need to stock anything more than simple airway devices such as oral or nasal airways unless you are planning (and have the skills) to give an anaesthetic for the simple reason that anyone one who requires advanced airway management is likely to be unsalvageable in an austere situation. If simple devices are not sufficient then they are likely to die regardless and introducing relatively complicated airway devices will not help. This, however, is an individual decision.

Contents

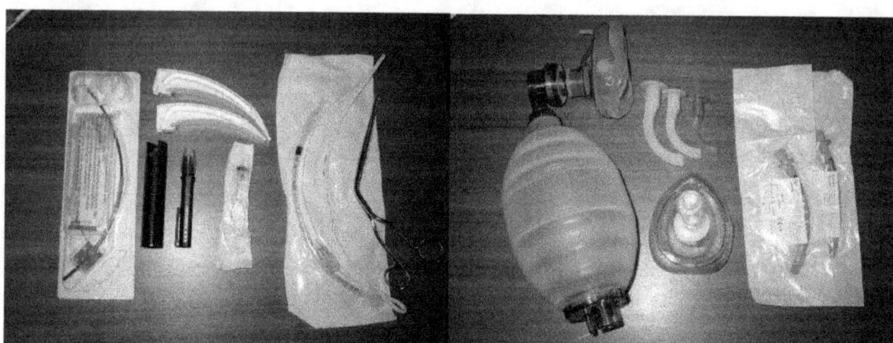

Figure 4.3 Basic airway equipment. From left – Surgical airway, Laryngoscope and blades, endotracheal tube, McGill forceps, self in ating bag and mask, oral and nasal airways.

First Aid Kit

A comprehensive basic first aid kit is the building block of any medical preparations. With relatively simple equipment and supplies you can stop bleeding, splint a fracture, and provide basic patient assessment. Table 4.1 lists the suggested contents for a basic first air kit. The following are the key components of any kit albeit for a work, sport, or survival orientated first aid kit:

Dressings – Small gauze squares/large squares/Combined dressings/battle dressings/ non-adhesive dressings. There is a vast range. They serve two functions: - to cover and stop bleeding and to protect a wound. Exactly what you need is to a large degree personal preference – but whatever you buy you need small and large sizes, and they need to be absorbent.

Roller/Crepe Bandages – These go by various names (Crepe, Kerlix) – but we are talking about is some form of elasticised roller bandage. These are required to hold dressings in place, apply pressure to bleeding wounds, to help splint fractures, and to strap and support joint sprains. They come in a variety of sizes from 3 cm to 15 cm (1- 4") and you should stock a variety of sizes

Triangular bandages – These are triangular shapes of material which can be used for making slings, and splinting fractures, and sprains.

Band-Aids – Lots of them and in multiple sizes. They are useful for protecting minor wounds and skin damage.

Oral or nasal airways and a CPR face shield – We have already discussed supplies for airway management. Oral or nasal airways are the basics for assisting with airway management. Often when combined with basic airway opening manoeuvres these are sufficient to maintain the airway of an unconscious person. The face shield is if you need to perform mouth-to-mouth on someone. This only really an issue with strangers not close friends or family members.

Contents

Sterile normal saline (salt water) or water – You don't need expensive antiseptic solutions for cleaning wounds. Sterile saline or water (and to be honest – even tap water is fine for most wound cleaning) is all that's required to irrigate or clean contaminated wounds. There is no clear evidence that using antiseptics over sterile water in traumatic (as opposed to surgical) cuts or abrasions reduces the incidence of infection. The best way to clean a wound is with copious amounts of water or saline. It is also useful for irrigating eyes which have been exposed to chemical, dust, or other foreign bodies.

Tape – You can never have too much tape. It has 100s of uses. We recommend a strong sticky tape like Sleek™ or Elastoplast™. There are many other paper or plastic based tapes around – the main criterion is that it always sticks when required.

Gloves – Needed for two reasons. Firstly you have to assume that everyone you deal with has a blood borne disease. When you are dealing with family members in an austere situation this isn't so important. The second reason is to try and reduce

infection when dealing with wounds. In the same way that using antiseptics over sterile water for irrigation of wounds has minimal impact on the incidence of infection

– the same is true for sterile vs. non-sterile gloves. When managing traumatic wounds (again this isn't true for surgical incisions and operations) there appears to be minimal difference in infection rates between wound management with sterile or non-sterile gloves. Exam gloves are not sterile, can be used on either hand, and are just casually sized (small, medium, large, etc.). They come in boxes of 50 or 100. Nitrile gloves are more than latex. Sterile gloves are packed individually and have specific sizes – 7.0, 7.5, 8.0, etc. Size is important – know your size.

That's it really, a very basic and limited range of supplies. As you can see this is considerably less than what is sold in many commercial first air kits but this is all that is required in a basic first aid kit. These supplies cover most first aid situations. They give you the ability to provide basic airway management, clean a wound, control bleeding, and splint, and immobilise fractures and sprains. It will also protect yourself from contamination with the gloves and face shield.

Basic Medical Kit

The basic medical kit is the next step you take from a basic first aid kit. The example here is designed for someone with a basic medical knowledge and a couple of good books. A lot of common problems can be managed with it; minor trauma (cuts and minor fractures), simple infections, and medical problems. Between this and the larger more comprehensive advanced kit wide spectrum dependent on knowledge or experience. Most begin with a first aid kit and expand as knowledge and finances allow.

A smaller medical kit for your bug-out bag could be made up from the above by adding some medications (such as acetaminophen, Benadryl, and some loperimide) and some instruments to a small first aid kit.

Advanced Medical kit

Contents

This is designed for someone with extensive medical training and would allow one to cope with 90% of common medical problems including some surgery, spinal and regional anaesthesia, and general anaesthesia with ketamine, treating most common infections and medical problems, and moderate trauma. This list may seem extreme, but is designed for a well-trained person in a worst-case scenario. Even though it is a long list, it all packs down. This sort of amount of equipment packs into two medium size nylon multi-compartment bags and a Plano rigid 747 box

Table 4.1 Basic First Aid Kit

Bandages and Dressings:

Antiseptic Wipes

Bandage (Crepe) – 50 mm (2")

Bandage (Crepe) – 75 mm (2.5")

Bandage (Crepe) – 100 mm (4")

Bandage (Gauze) – 75 mm (2.5")

Bandage (Gauze) – 100 mm (4") Bandage Triangular

Dressing (Combine) 90 mm x 100 m m Dressing (Combine) 200 mm x 200 mm Dressing (Non Adhesive) 75 mm x 50 mm Dressing (Non Adhesive) 75 mm x 100 mm Dressing Strip - Elastoplast 75 mm x 1 m Eye Pads

Gauze Swabs (Pkt 2) – 100 mm x 100 mm Sticking plasters

Personal protection

Disposable Gloves CPR Face Shield

Instruments

Clothing Shears Tweezers - Fine Point Splinter Probes

Other

Contents

Saline Solution 30 mL Tubes Steri-Strips – 3 mm

Survival Sheet Tape – 25 mm

Table 4.2. Basic medical kit

Bandages and Dressings

Combat Dressings Large gauze dressings Small gauze squares

Roller Bandages elastic + cotton (2in/4in/6in) Triangular Bandages

Bandaids -assorted sizes and shapes (i.e. finger tips) Sleek Tape 1 in. (waterproof, plastic/elasticised tape) Cotton buds (Q-tips, cotton tips)

Personal protection / Antisepsis:

Chlorhexidine (Hibiclens) or Povidone-iodine (Disinfectant) Antibacterial Soap

Gloves

Saline solution – for irrigation

Medication:

Lignocaine 1% (Lidocaine) Augmentin Acetaminophen (Tylenol) Diclophenac (Voltaren) Oral Rehydration powder Loperamide (Imodium) Benadryl &/or Claritin

(local anaesthetic)

(broad spectrum antibiotic) (mild analgesic)

(mod analgesic/antiinflammatory)

(antidiarrhoeal)

(antihistamines, short + long acting)

Contents

Adrenaline auto injector (Epicene) (USA = epinephrine) Morphine Sulphate (strong pain killer) if available Gamma Benzene Hexachloride (lice/scabies treatment)

Co-timoxazole (antifungal) Contraceptive pills/Condoms

Instruments:

Clothing shears

Surgical scissors)

Needle holder) Sm curved clamps) Tissue forceps)

Scalpel blades)

Enough to do basic minor surgery - suturing, draining abscesses, cleaning a wound, etc.

Other:

Thermometer (rectal or pacifier for children) Emergency Obstetric Kit (includes bulb suction)

Vicryl 2-0 suture material

(Your choice of suture material is up to you – and is covered in detail elsewhere in this book. Vicryl is a synthetic dissolvable one, but takes up to 4-6 weeks to dissolve, so I think it is the ideal survival thread)

5 mL syringes

20 gauge needles

Dental:

Oil of cloves

(tooth ache)

Emergency dental kit (commercial preparation)

Contents

Contents

Contents

Emergency Obstetric Kit (includes cord clamps, bulb suction etc) Suture Material Vicryl; 0, 2-0

Chromic 0, 2-0

Dermalon 0, 2-0 Surgical stapler and remover

Heimlich flutter valve Chest drains – various sizes

Drainage bottles or Flutter valves Penrose drains

Foley Urethral Catheters – 16 French (most useful size) Urine Bags

Nasogastric (NG) tubes + spigots Heavy duty scissors

Medications

Povidone - iodine Prep antiseptic skin prep and/or

Alcohol prep antiseptic skin prep

Chlorhexidine and cetrimide antiseptic hand wash

Benalkium Chloride Antirabies skin wash Antibacterial Soap

Paracetamol (Tylenol) oral mild analgesic Aspirin oral wonder drug

Diclophenac oral mod analgesic (NASID)

Morphine IV/IMSC strong analgesic

Naroxone IV antagonist to morphine

Ketamine IV/IM IV anaesthetic

Diazepam IV hypnotic/sedative

Contents

Surgical Instruments

Contents

The above kits are general medical kits – covering the multitude of medical problems and contain surgical instruments. However commonly asked questions relate specifically to surgical instruments – what and how many of them are required for various levels of surgical procedures. Below is a detailed list of surgical instruments with 4 levels of increasing complexity. Note that each level builds on the one before it. This instrument list reflects our own preferences and experience under austere conditions. There are many other instruments that would be helpful (for example ring forceps to hold sponges, larger retractors, etc.), but they are not considered vital. This is the bare minimum.

What is it?

Needle holders – shaped like scissors but instead of having a cutting surface they have two opposed plates with groves cut into them, and are designed to hold the needle, and stop it rolling or slipping as you sew. Once you have gripped the needle a ratchet holds the tips locked so the needle does not move

Haemostat/Clips/Clamps – Similar in shape to needle holders but the tips are designed to clamp onto tissue and to hold it. They have the same ratchet mechanism to keep them locked and attached once they are attached. They are used to clip bleeding blood vessels or hold onto tissues you are working with. There is a massive range of sizes and shapes depending on what they are designed to clip or clamp.

Forceps/Dissectors – are shaped like traditional tweezers and come in various sizes. They either have small teeth on their tips or are smooth tipped. They are designed to handle tissues and to help you move tissues round such as when suturing

Scissors – these are self-explanatory

Retractors – these are designed to hold tissues out of the way so that you can see what you are doing. They come in a huge range of sizes and shapes depending on what part of the body you are working with. Skin hooks or small right-angle retractors are most suitable for most minor wound repairs

Level 1: Field Wound Repair Kit

This is a minimal cost unit intended to be carried in a kit or pack, and be used for minor wound debridement, and closure of the types of injuries most commonly occurring. Although it is a pre-packaged "disposable" kit the instruments may be reused many times with appropriate sterilization and care. This easily goes in a zip- lock bag, and can be widely distributed, and available among your group.

Level 2: Basic Suture Tray

This is composed of good quality instruments intended for long term use and resterilization. It is suitable for repair and debridement of minor wounds and injuries including simple two-layer closure. This is typical of the majority of wound care done in a hospital ER.

Contents

Level 3: Procedure kit

This kit is capable of complicated multilayer wound repair, OB repairs, plastic surgery closures, tendon repair, chest tube insertion. This is suitable for laymen with some training and experience, and is probably the recommended level for most as it has the greatest capability vs. expense. Those with adequate medical training could press this into service for more advanced problems with some improvisation.

Note: if you anticipate a lot of OB or foreign body removal a Weitlaner retractor, 5-6" would be very helpful. A rongeur and rasp are very helpful for bone clean up, traumatic finger amputations, etc.

Level 4: Major procedures kit

This kit is capable of complicated multilayer wound repair, OB repairs, plastic surgery closures, tendon repair, chest tube insertion, emergency abdominal surgery, Caesarean sections, straightforward amputations, etc. With this kit a competent practitioner should be able to perform all the procedures that are likely to be possible in an austere environment.

Table 4.4 Field Wound repair kit

1

1

1

1

1

Tube Super-glue Gel

Steri-Strips, and Benzoin adhesive, or duct tape Betadine swab packet, or skin cleaner of choice

Irrigation syringe and ability to purify at least 2 quarts water; tablets, etc. Dressings of choice

Optional items to consider include:

1

Contents

Disposable laceration tray with needle driver, pick-ups, scissors, 4x4s, drape Disposable scalpel, #10

Ethilon, or Prolene, or Silk 4-0 & 6-0 Vicryl or Chromic 4-0

skin stapler, 15 shot staple remover

Sterile gloves your size

Lidocaine 1% or 2% WITHOUT epinephrine

Table 4.5 Basic suture tray

Contents

Needle driver, 5"

Adson forceps ,1x2 teeth Sharp/blunt scissors, 5" straight Iris tissue scissors, curved Mosquito hemostat, curved

#3 Scalpel handle & #10, #11, #15 blades

Ethilon, or Prolene, or Silk suture; 2-0, 4-0, 6-0, cuticular needles Vicryl or Chromic suture 2-0, 4-0, 6-0 cuticular needles

Skin staplers & remover Steri-Strips and Benzoin Several tubes Super-glue Gel Skin cleaner of choice

Irrigation syringes & ability to purify water Sterile gloves appropriate sizes

Sterile drapes, disposable or reusable Appropriate anaesthesia and dressing of choice

Table 4.6 Procedure set

1

1

1

1

1

1

1

1

1

1

1

Contents

Contents

Steri-Strips and Benzoin Several tubes Super-glue Gel Skin cleaner of choice

Irrigation syringes & ability to purify water Sterile gloves appropriate sizes

Sterile drapes, disposable or reusable Appropriate anaesthesia and dressing of choice

Table 4.7 Major Procedure kit

1

1

1

2

1

1

1

1

1

2

2

2

1

1

1

Contents

Needle driver, 4-5"

Needle driver, 6-7"

Sharp/blunt scissors, 5" straight

Baby Metzenbaum or Mayo scissors, 5" curved Metzenbaum, 6-7" Curved

Mayo, 6-7" Curved

Iris tissue scissors, curved Mosquito haemostat, straight Mosquito haemostat, curved Kelly haemostat, straight Kelly haemostat, curved

Contents

Chapter 5 Antibiotics

Antibiotics are one of the most talked about subjects in austere and survival medicine. This is an area where there is widespread misinformation and ignorance. There are multiple different antibiotics and they work best depending on the bacteria causing the infection and the location of the infection. What follows is an overview designed to give you a better understanding of what works for what.

Antibiotics only work in bacterial infections and some parasitic infections. They don't work in treating viral infections which accounts for the vast majority of coughs, colds, flu's, earache, sinus, and chest infections which people suffer from every winter.

Contents

While there are some specific antiviral medications most viruses do not have a specific drug to treat infections caused by them.

There is no one antibiotic that works in every situation and giving the wrong antibiotic can be worse (long-term) than not giving one at all. Each organism has one or two antibiotics that are specific for that organism and that is the antibiotic which should be used.

The Bacteria:

A basic understanding of how bugs (read bacteria) cause infections is required to appropriately use antibiotics. There are hundreds of millions of different species of bacteria; most do not cause illness in man.

There are four main classes of bacteria

- Gram-positive (+ ve)
- Gram-negative (- ve)
- Anaerobes
- Others

Gram-positive bacteria stain blue and gram-negative bacteria stain pink when subjected to a gram staining test. They are further subdivided by their shape (cocci = round, bacilli = oval) and if they form aggregates or not. This is described in much more detail in chapter 8. Anaerobic bacteria are ones which require no oxygen to grow.

Gram-Positive Bacteria (Gram +ve)

Contents

- Staphylococcus: Commonest pathogen is S. aureus; Gram-positive cocci in clumps. Causes boils, abscesses, impetigo, wound infections, bone infections, pneumonia (uncommonly), food poisoning, and septicaemia. Generally very sensitive to Flucloxacillin as first choice drug, and Augmentin, and the cephalosporins. A strain which is resistant to the above known as MRSA is currently treated with vancomycin.
- Streptococcus: Gram-positive cocci in pairs or chains. Most are not pathogenic in man except Strep pneumoniae and the Strep pyogenes. Strep pneumoniae causes pneumonia, ear infections, sinusitis, meningitis, septic arthritis, and bone infections. Strep pyogenes causes sore throats, impetigo, scarlet fever, cellulitis, septicaemia, and necrotising fasciitis. Streps are usually very sensitive to penicillins, cephalosporins, and the quinolones.

Gram-Negative Bacteria (Gram -ve)

Neisseria meningitidis: Gram-negative cocci in pairs. Common cause of bacterial meningitis, may also cause pneumonia and septicaemia. Can be rapidly fatal.

Sensitive to penicillins, cephalosporins, quinolones, Co-trimoxazole, and tetracyclines.

Contents

- Neisseria gonorrhoeae: Gram-negative cocci in pairs. Causes gonorrhoea. Sensitive to high dose amoxicillin (single dose), Augmentin, and also cephalosporins, and quinolones.
- Moxella catarrhalis: Gram-negative cocci in pairs. Common cause of ear and sinus infections, also chronic bronchitis exacerbations. Sensitive to Augmentin, cephalosporins, quinolones, Co-trimoxazole, and tetracyclines.
- Haemophilus influenzae: Gram-negative cocci-bacilli. Can cause meningitis (esp. in children under 5), epiglottitis, cellulitis, and a sub group causes chest infections. Sensitive as M.catarrhalis
- Escherichia coli: Gram-negative bacilli. Normally found in the bowel. Causes urinary infections, severe gastroenteritis, peritonitis (from bowel injury), and septicaemia. The antibiotic of choice has traditionally been a quinolone or cephalosporin. However E.Coli is becoming increasingly resistant to both (although in many areas they work fine – that is why it is important to understand local resistant patterns which can be obtained from the microbiology labs at your local hospital).We recommend Co-trimoxazole as a first choice – especially for urinary tract infections.
- Proteus species (sp).: Gram-negative bacilli. Lives in the bowel. Causes Urinary tract infections (UTI's), peritonitis (from bowel injuries), and wound infections. Drug of choice is the quinolones.

Anaerobes

Contents

- Bacteroides sp.: Gram-negative bacilli. Normal bowel flora. Commonly causes infections following injury to the bowel, or wound contamination, causes abscess formation. Treated first choice with metronidazole or second with chloramphenicol or Augmentin. Chloramphenicol is moderately high risk with high doses (>4gm/day) causing bone marrow suppression which rarely can be fatal – but it is cheap, readily available, and complications are rare. Metronidazole and cefotaxime IV combination is good for Bacteroides fragilis. Zosyn or imipenem is a good single agent therapy.
- Clostridium sp.: Gram-positive species produce spores and toxins:

  1. C. perfringens/C. septicum - common cause of gangrene; treat with penicillins or metronidazole
  2. C. tetani - tetanus damage is from toxins, not the bacteria themselves.
  3. C. botulinum - botulism)
  4. C. difficille - causes diarrhoea following antibiotic dosages; treat with metronidazole

Others:

- Chlamydia sp: Includes C. pneumonia; responsible for a type of atypical pneumonia and C. trachomatis; responsible for the sexually transmitted disease Chlamydia. It is best treated with tetracyclines or as second choice a macrolide.
- Mycoplasma pneumoniae: A cause of atypical pneumonia. Treated best with a macrolide, second choice of tetracycline.

Antibiotics

Penicillins - These act by preventing replicating bacteria from producing a cell wall. A number of bacteria produce an enzyme which inactivates the penicillins (B- lactamase).

A number of varieties:

Contents

- Benzylpenicillin (Penicillin G Benzathine): Injectable preparation. Antibiotic of choice against severe Strep pneumoniae and Neisseria sp infections such as chest infections, meningitis, and cellulitis.
- Phenoxymethyl penicillin (Penicillin V): Oral preparation of above. Usually used only for the treatment of sore throats (strep throats); in other infections largely replaced by amoxicillin which is better absorbed.
- Flucloxacillin: Oral and IV drug of choice for Staph infection such as cellulitis, boils, abscess, and bone infections. Also usually effective against Strep but not first choice.
- Amoxicillin: (newer version of ampicillin): Oral and IV. Effective against most gram-positive and negative bugs. Limited use secondary to B-lactamase resistance in many bugs. Beta-lactamase production is a method by which the bacteria try and protect themselves against an antibiotic – it is a bacterial enzyme which breaks down the main active ingredient of penicillin antibiotics. This is overcome with the addition of clavulanic acid (e.g. Augmentin). Overcoming this resistance makes this combination my ideal survival antibiotic, with good gram-positive, negative, and

anaerobic cover. This drug we feel is the best broad-spectrum antibiotic commonly available. Other antibiotics may be better for specific infections but this is the best all purpose one.

Cephalosporins - Same method of action as penicillins. Developed in three generations. There is now a fourth but not yet widely available. The third generation e.g., efotaxime (Claforan, IV only) and ceftriaxone (Rocephin, IV/IM only) have the most broad spectrum effect. They are effective against most gram-positives, negatives, and some variable anaerobic cover. The second generation e.g., cefuroxime (Zinacef, oral and IV) and Cefaclor (Ceclor, oral only) also have good general coverage, but are

not as effective against some gram-negative bacilli. This loss of gram-negative coverage expands to most gram-negative cocci and bacilli in the first-generation cephalosporins e.g., cephalexin (Ke ex, oral only) and cephazolin (Kefzol, IV only). The third generation is ideal for use in those with very severe generalised infection, meningitis, or intra-abdominal sepsis (e.g., penetrating abdominal wound or appendicitis), with metronidazole added in, and the second-generation offers a good broad-spectrum antibiotic for general use in skin, wound, urinary, and chest infections.

Contents

Quinolones - Act by inhibiting DNA replication in the nucleus of the replicating bacteria. This is a new generation of antibiotics. Most common is ciprofloxacin. They offer very broad spectrum cover except for anaerobes. Excellent survival antibiotic and our second choice due to the fact that amoxycillin + clavulanic acid gives better cover of anaerobes. Effective for most types of infections except intra- abdominal sepsis and gangrene.

Gatifloxacin (Tequin) is recommended by the TCCC for gunshot or fragment wounds. It is very broad spectrum and has once daily dosing. It is relatively expensive at about

$10 USD a tablet

Macrolides - Act by inhibiting protein synthesis in the replicating bacteria. Includes erythromycin, and the newer Roxithromycin, and clarithromycin. Often used for people with a penicillin allergy, however it does have a reduced spectrum (esp. with gram-negatives) but is an alternative to tetracycline in Chlamydia. First choice in atypical pneumonias, e.g. with Mycoplasma pneumonia.

Co-trimoxazole (SMX-TMP) - Acts by interfering with folate metabolism in the replicating bacteria. Previously a very broad-spectrum antibiotic now has a much more variable response rate due to resistance. Still useful for urinary and mild chest infections.

Tetracyclines – Acts by blocking protein synthesis. Broad-spectrum coverage – gram-positive, gram-negative, anaerobes; rickettsiae (syphilis, typhus), Chlamydia, and Mycoplasma. A commonly used treatment for common biological warfare agents

– Anthrax, Tularaemia, Plague, Brucellosis, Melioidosis, Psittacosis, Q fever, Typhus. Good oral absorption. Can be given parentally – but commercial preparations now uncommon. Can cause bone and teeth growth problems when given to children. As discussed elsewhere used to be manufactured with a compound which became toxic as it broke down – this no longer occurs.

Metronidazole (Flagyl) - Acts by directly damaging the structure of the DNA of the bacteria/protozoa. Drug of choice for anaerobic infection. Should be used with another broad-spectrum antibiotic for any one with possible faecal contamination of a wound or intra-abdominal sepsis (such as severe appendicitis). Also the drug of choice for parasitic infections such as Giardia.

In the same family as Metronidazole is tinidazole (Fasigyn). The treatment course is usually shorter with generally less side effects and is cheaper. It is also more effective against Giardia.

Others - There are many other antibiotics available. We have only discussed the common ones above.

For further information you should consult any major antibiotic guide (see Reference Books chapter). Which bacteria are sensitive to which antibiotics varies to a degree depending on local resistance patterns among the bacteria – local hospitals will normally be able to tell you what the local patterns are for common bacteria

Contents

In pregnancy penicillins and cephalosporins are safe to use. Many others are not (or only during certain parts of the pregnancy). You should always check if any drug you are using is safe, before using in pregnancy and breast-feeding. The PDR will tell you. If you want a specific reference try "Drugs in Pregnancy", Ed D.F. Hawkins.

Chapter 6 Sterilisation and Disinfection

Throughout this book we have tried to emphasize the importance of basic hygiene in any survival situation. This is especially true when performing any surgical procedure

- from suturing a small cut or dressing a wound, to dealing with a major injury or performing an operation.

Cleaning, Disinfection, and Sterilization of medical instruments and supplies

Q. What is the difference between disinfection and sterilization?

A. An item is sterile when it is made completely free of measurable levels of microorganisms (bacteria, viruses, fungal spores) by a chemical or physical process of sterilization. Disinfection describes the process of destroying microorganisms or inhibiting their growth but is generally less absolute. All sterile items are disinfected but not all disinfected items are sterile. In some cases disinfection removes most but not all of the microbes, or removes all bacteria but not fungal spores, etc.

Sterility is only a temporary state – once sterile packaging is open or the product has been removed from an autoclave colonization begins almost immediately just from exposure to air and bacteria present in the environment.

Q. What is the difference between clean and sterile?

A. We have defined sterile above; clean is the absence of dirt. It is possible to have an item which is dirty yet sterile, i.e. the dirt is sterile. The gold standard is clean AND sterile. That said sterility is over-rated to a point. Clean items are sufficient to prevent infection in the majority of cases. Sterility is required when you are invading the body cavities or deep tissues. For the vast majority of minor cuts and lacerations clean is fine. Bulk unsterilised gauze is much cheaper than the same amount of sterile material.

Infection rates are no greater if a superficial wound has been irrigated and cleaned with tap water vs. being cleaned and irrigated with sterile saline. The studies supporting this are based on municipal tap water supply – so is not completely applicable to all situations.

Expendable vs. Reusable:

Contents

Expendable supplies are used once and discarded. You will eventually run out of them no matter how much you have stored. They also create a medical waste problem and that waste can spread disease. Reusable supplies are just that, they last longer but not forever. Whenever possible use a reusable item.

Sterilisation of specific items:

In this section we discuss what methods can be used for different items or categories of medical consumables and any caveats related to specific types of material you should be aware of. The following sections will deal specifically with how to do the actual disinfection or sterilising.

Syringes:

There are two types of syringes: disposable and reusable. The main differences relate to the material used to make the barrel and plunger of the syringe. A reusable syringe's body and plunger will either be made of glass or a plastic that can be autoclaved. The rubber on a "reusable" plastic plunger will break down with autoclaving or the glazing on the glass plunger will eventually wear out. Again, permanent supplies are not forever.

Reusable needles will generally have a Luer lock attachment to attach to the syringe (as do many disposable ones) and will be made of a harder metal so they can be re- sharpened. They will also come with a needle plunger so anything trapped in the needle cylinder can be removed.

Disposable syringes will generally melt when heated to sterilising temperatures but can be autoclaved several times before deforming beyond usefulness.

Contemporary practice is that diabetics using syringes to administer their insulin can reuse the same syringe for up to a week (SQ injections) if kept in a clean container and there is no need to sterilize them within this period. This could be extrapolated to reusing the same syringe when administering a series of injections of the same medication to the same person over a short-term period in an austere situation (SOLELY to the same person).

The best method to sterilise syringes is to use a rack to suspend the barrel and plunger. The WHO has reported a 40% failure rate with other methods. A large part of this failure rate is thought to be due to laying the components in a tray. Any points of contact with a tray are areas the steam or heat cannot get to, so it's partially insulated, and some organisms may survive.

A rack should be made of metal and constructed so that the syringe bodies, plungers, and needles can be suspended in them with minimal contact with the rack itself so as to be hanging relatively freely. Racks can be easily made at home.

If you don't have a rack an alternate method is to wrap the plunger and cylinder in an OR towel and push the needles through the cloth. Nothing should be in contact with each other. Fold to make a pack and autoclave.

Contents

If you do not have access to a pressure cooker or autoclave boiling is acceptable but a distant second choice.

The type of water used in an autoclave or pressure cooker will probably effect the life

span of permanent syringes – the harder the water the less reuses – a very rough guide is: hard water = 50-60 reuses, soft water = 200+ reuses. It is impossible to say with certainty how long a glass syringe will last. Using hard water may also create maintenance problems for a pressure cooker although many home canners have used hard water for years with minimal problems.

Sharpening permanent needles:

Place a drop of light oil (sewing machine, light machine, or gun oil) on a fine sharpening stone. Draw the bevel (flat part of tip) of the needle back and forth at a uniform angle with no rocking. The goal is to keep the bevel the same length as on a new needle. Any rocking side to side will cause the bevel to become rounded and must be corrected. Rocking the angle of attack against the stone will cause at best, a dull needle and at worst a hook on the point.

After sharpening for a bit a burr will form on the sides of the bevel – this is a thin edge of metal. Remove it by gently drawing the needle on the side, to the top – forming 2 facets along the top of the point.

Always finish by giving one rub along the bevel and one to each facet.

When finished, check with a magnifying glass. Needles should be soaked

overnight in trichloroethylene to remove any oil then polished with a soft cloth and water pushed through them to make sure the cylinder is clear

If you do not have access to oil and a solvent to remove it, then sharpen and clean (including inside the barrel – using fine wire) using hot soapy water.

This procedure should be done when the needle seems to be getting dull not after every use.

Section 12.10 of "A Medical Laboratory for Developing Countries" by Maurice King has slightly more complete instructions along with very good illustrations for this procedure.

Surgical instruments:

Contents

Options for sterilizing instruments in order of preference are: Pressure cooker or autoclave, oven (may damage instruments over time leading to cracks and possible breakage), isopropyl flaming (doesn't kill everything and eventually damages metal), and heating to red hot and letting cool (kills everything but damages metal - emergency use only), chemical soaking (generally doesn't kill everything), and boiling.

Instruments with opposing surfaces (scissors, clips) should be sterilized open. There is a risk of sharp edge rust - wrap scalpel blades and individual scissor blades in a piece of paper with a single fold this serves to wick moisture away and prevent rust.

The paper can be reused and in the case of scalpel blades used as a storage container for the blades.

Scalpel blades and scissors can be sharpened with a fine stone. Metal instruments with moving parts can be lubricated with light machine oil or gun oil. Stainless steel can rust if the finish is scratched so should be handled with care. Sterilizing an instrument that has started to rust with those that have not will cause the rust to spread.

Dressings and other textiles:

Autoclave/Pressure cook.

Disinfection can be accomplished with the following methods:

- Ironing on a table covered with a drape that has been ironed and dampen each item with boiled water. The iron should be hot and several passes made.
- Hanging in full sunlight for 6 hours per side.
- Wash and boil for 5 minutes.
- Wash, rinse, and soak for 30 minutes in a 0.1% chlorine solution or 5% Lysol solution.

Gloves, tubing, and other rubber items:

Autoclave/Pressure Cook. Blow into the gloves to ensure no leaks; if leaks patch from the inside. Powder all rubber items with talcum powder prior to sterilizing and thoroughly let dry before storing or they will stick together. Repeated autoclaving will break down rubber.

Plastic Items (airways, syringes, etc):

The correct method depends on the plastic used in the manufacture and this may be difficult to discover.

Contents

HDPE (High Density Polyethylene): Translucent. Autoclave at 121 C for no more than 15 min.

PP (Polypropylene): Translucent. Autoclave at 121 C

PMP (Polymethylpentene): Clear. Brittle at room temp, can crack or break if dropped. Autoclave at 121 C.

PC (Polycarbonate): Clear. Autoclave at 121 C.

PTFE (Polytetrafluoroethylene): Not translucent. Autoclave at 121 C or oven at 160 C (320 F) for 2 hours or 170 C (340 F) for 1 hour.

Glassware:

Autoclave/Pressure cook

Glassware can crack or shatter if the autoclave or pressure cooker is opened too soon. Pipettes may not fit in a pressure cooker.

Culture media:

Autoclave/Pressure cook.

It will boil and spatter if the pressure cooker is opened too soon. Shelf life of prepared media:

Tubes with cotton-wool plugs – 3 weeks Tubes with loose caps – 2 weeks Containers with screw caps – 3 months

Petri dishes (if sealed in plastic bags) – 4 weeks

Preparation of Distilled Water:

Distilled water is the preferred type of water for use in autoclaves and pressure cookers for sterilisation. Sterile distilled water is also the preferred type for the production of IV fluids, and wound cleaning, and irrigation. Distilled water is sterilised by boiling.

Options:

Contents

Snow and rain: Freshly fallen snow and rain are good sources as long as you are not in a city due to the high risk of contamination of city air. For snow use the top layer only. If you don't get to it right after it starts snowing, scrape off the top layer, and collect underlying layers avoiding the bottom layers. Once melted this can be considered the equivalent of distilled water.

Streams, springs, and wells: Most springs, streams, and all rivers in US are contaminated to varying degrees be it with commercial effluent, or natural mineral run-off, or animal faeces. Being safe to drink – which many streams in wilderness areas are, is not the same as being nearly distilled in quality. The conditions in other countries vary but those close to the equator can host more lethal or harmful organisms due to environmental factors. Wells are usually relatively uncontaminated with micro-organisms but they frequently will have a high mineral content and should be distilled before use in a pressure cooker.

Filtration: Commercial water filters do not produce pure distilled quality water but it is close; depending on the type of filter they remove bacteria, viruses, parasites, heavy metals, and some other chemicals. Ceramic water filters can be scrubbed and reused.

Distilling water: The simplest method for distilling water is using the FEMA method. A large pot with a lid is filled 1/3 to 1/2 full of water. The lid is inverted and a coat hanger or wire is used to suspend a right side up coffee cup under the inverted handle. Steam collects on the pot lid and drips down the handle into the coffee cup when the pot is boiled. Let it cool and collect the distilled water in the cup. The less water boiled the less fuel used, but the closer the pot has to be watched.

Preparation of water for drinking

The methods described above to produce distilled water will generally produce water of good enough quality for drinking. We do not cover in detail water purification for drinking, but due to the fact chemical disinfection is a regular question in survival medicine forums here is an overview:

Chemical disinfection of water for drinking:

For chemical disinfection, the key is the concentration of halogenation:

Contents

Concentration of Halogen	Contact time @ 5°C / 41° F	Contact time @ 15° C / 59° F	Contact time @ 30° C / 86° F
2 ppm	240 minutes	180 minutes	60 minutes
4 ppm	180 min	60 min	45 min
8 ppm	60 min	30 min	15 min

Per liter of water, Iodine tabs (tetraglycine hydroperiodide, EDWGT (emergency drinking water germicidal tablets), Potable Aqua (trade name), Globaline (trade name)

:

4 ppm – ½ tab 8 ppm – 1 tab

These tablets should be gunmetal grey in color when used – if rust colored they are useless: The free iodine has combined with atmospheric moisture. The bottles should be kept well sealed and replaced often.

Contents

2% iodine (tincture of Iodine)	4 ppm – 0.2 ml (5 gtts)	8 ppm – 0.4 ml (10 gtts)
10% povidone-iodine (Betadine)	4 ppm - 0.35 ml (8 gtts)	8 ppm – 0.7ml (16 gtts)
solution only, NOT SCRUB		
Saturated iodine crystals	4 ppm – 13 ml	8 ppm – 26 ml
Iodine crystals in alcohol	0.1 ml / 5 ppm	0.2 ml / 10 ppm
Halazone Monodichloroaminobenzoic acid tablets	4 ppm – 2 tabs	8 ppm – 4 tabs
Household bleach (Clorox)	4 ppm – 0.1 ml (2 gtts)	8 ppm – 0.2 ml (4 gtts)

For very cold water contact time should be increased.

If drinking this water after disinfection, flavouring agents (drink mixes, etc) can be added: This must be done AFTER the period allocated for disinfection (the disinfecting agent will bind to the organic material and not work).

This information is taken from the Wilderness Medical Society Practice Guidelines 2nd Edition, edited by William Forgey MD (page 63)

Methods of disinfecting and sterilizing

Contents

Preparing materials to sterilise:

Contaminated materials should be disinfected prior to cleaning and sterilising. The point of this step is to kill any dangerous organisms (such as hepatitis B or C) and make them safer to clean. To do this place in a pressure cooker and bring to pressure then cook for 5 minutes. Alternatively, materials can be soaked in a chemical disinfectant for 30 minutes, then rinsed in cold water, and dried.

Once disinfected proceed with any additional maintenance, cleaning, and making up into packs. Disinfection can be skipped if dangerous organisms are not an issue. Initial rinsing with cold water to dislodge any organic matter is recommended to avoid coagulation.

Packs can be wrapped in paper (Kraft, newspaper, etc.) and/or a tightly woven textile. A double wrap is ideal for a shelf life of several weeks. Using autoclave bags will result in much longer shelf life but these are not really reusable. An ideal wrap would be a layer of cloth inside and paper outside.

Thermal

Boiling in water: Boil in water for 20-30 minutes (at sea level). In theory the time should be increased by 5 minutes for each 1,000 ft rise in altitude, however, in practice this will have a minimal impact on sterility (the vast majority of pathogenic organisms are killed at temperatures of > 85 degrees C for several minutes) and simply wastes fuel. If your instruments where grossly contaminated by the previous patient - using these adjustments may be appropriate. The addition of 2% sodium carbonate will increase the effectiveness of the process.

Boiling will cause rusting of anything that holds an edge such as scissors and knives. Using distilled or soft water will reduce this problem. Do not start timing until the water has come to a full boil. Note that boiling will not kill spores but will kill HIV and hepatitis B.

Consider vacuum packing items in "boil in bag" pouches – this will enable them to be sterilised and protect against rusting.

Oven: 160 C (320 F) for 2 hours or 170 C (340 F) for 1 hour (Do not exceed 170 C or metal instruments may be damaged). Leave oven door open the first few minutes of heating to vacate any moisture and prevent rusting of metal items, and do not start timing till the desired temperature has been reached. This method is acceptable for surgical instruments, and high temperature glass, or plastics but not for textiles. Oils, ointments, waxes, and powders should be heated at 160 C (320 F) for 2 hours.

Solar - for textiles, hanging in full sun and fresh air for 6 hours per side will disinfect.

Ironing - for textiles heat the iron very hot and lay the textile on another textile that has itself been ironed. Steam lightly and make several slow passes with the iron.

Contents

Flaming

1. Alcohol – dip the instrument in alcohol and set fire to it. This method is not reliable and will damage instruments in the long term but is better than nothing.
2. Heating in open flame till red hot. This method is reliable but should be used in emergencies only as it WILL damage the instrument.

Using a pressure cooker as an autoclave

Care and feeding of pressure cookers: You should clean after each use with distilled water or fresh rainwater. Do not use detergents. Check the gasket, pressure vent, gauge, etc. You should check the manual which comes with your pressure

cooker for specifics on maintenance. The manual is perhaps the most important piece of equipment as specific pressure cookers vary somewhat in operation, inspection, and parts. The most important information in the manual will be time variations, how much water to add, and how to tell when it's safe to open it.

You should ensure you have spare parts, including a spare gasket (or two) and safety plug.

Packing: The internal packing needs to be loose so the steam can circulate around all the items. Don't mix loads of dissimilar items if at all possible.

TST test tape is an autoclave indicator tape. It changes colour when a load has been sterilised. It has a shelf life of 2 years from date of manufacture for

reliable results.

Operating: Bring the pressure cooker to full boil with the weight off or valve open. When it reaches a full boil (like a tea kettle telling you it's

ready - whistling) add weight or close valve and ONLY THEN begin timing. This is to evacuate all the air and replace it with steam.

If this is not done the needed temperature will not be reached and hostile organisms can survive.

Water: If possible use distilled or fresh rainwater. Hard water may cause layers of mineral deposits to build up and cause eventual failure if not cleaned regularly.

Enough water must be used so the pressure cooker does not run dry; if it does it can seriously damage the pressure cooker and potentially turn it into a bomb.

Contents

Time, pressure, and altitude: Do not begin timing until the pressure cooker is at full steam. You can test to see when all air is evacuated by attaching a rubber tube to the vent with the other end underwater. When bubbles stop coming up all air has been evacuated. Time this and in the future you can make sure the pressure cooker has this much "warm up" time before you start timing. Run at 121 C (250 F) for 30 minutes at 15 pounds pressure at sea level add 5 for every 500 ft gain in elevation. Use 40 minutes if cooking textiles.

Time and temp for culture media is different. Some media will experience shifts in pH or destruction of some components if over-autoclaved. You should consult the information that came with the media for specifics.

Cooling off: The time required to cool off is load dependent; glass (can shatter) and culture media (which can boil and spatter) take the longest cooling time. The latter can take several hours of cooling time . For other items allow at least 30 minutes for the pressure cooker to cool. Quick cooling is possible by running cold water over it – but with glass inside this increases the chance of shattering.

The drying of packs should be done by placing in a warm place on a rack.

Chemical:

Ethanol: You can ferment and distil your own although care needs to be taken so you don't produce toxic alcohols (e.g. methanol). Good for small cuts, surface preparation (including skin prep for surgery – toxic to deeper tissues and will sting ++), and instrument sterilisation. For instruments it is recommended that soaking in > 70% (ideal is >95%) solution for >12 hrs is ideal. This time can be shortened to several hours by the addition of formaldehyde solution to the alcohol.

Polyvidone-iodine (Betadine): There are some military reports of using to sterilise water for drinking. Exact details are scant. For soaking instruments 1 part 10% solution (Betadine) to 3 parts water for 15 min.

Hypochlorites (Clorox, etc) /bleach: 0.1% or 1,000 ppm. Bleach is useful for disinfecting surfaces and soaking instruments. Soak for 15 min but no longer than 30 min – bleach solutions are corrosive to metal instruments. The instruments should be rinsed upon removal from solution and dried. Production of bleach is described in Chapter 11: Long-Term Survival Medicine. Bleach breaks down relatively rapidly and most commercial solutions will have lost their active ingredients after 12-18 months.

Bleach in dilute concentrations can be used for wound care especially as a wash for burns. Start with a dilute concentration initially (1:60) if pain results from this concentration dilute it again by the same volume (out to 1:120), and increase the contact time.

Other chemical disinfectant agents:

Tosylchloramide Chloramine T 2% solution, 20g/litre for 15 min Ethanol 70%, 8 parts of 90% ethanol in 2 parts water for 15 min.

Isopropanol 70%, 7 parts isopropanol in 3 parts water for 15 min.

Formaldehyde 4%, 1 part formalin in 3 parts water for 30 min. Glutaraldehyde 2% add to supplied activator and soak for 30 min.

Other options:

Wines prepared from grapes may be useful as wound washes and antiseptics. If pain results from application of a small amount of wine to a wound the wine should be diluted using clean water until it can be applied without undue pain. The antiseptic effects of wine are due both to the ethanol present in the wine and to the presence

of some antibiotic materials. Grape juice may also be used with some effect. Some fruit wines also contain antibacterial agents.

Absent any other disinfectant or sterilising remember "the solution to pollution

is dilution;" wash the instruments with soap and copious amounts of water or lavage a wound with large amounts of water. When you need to repeatedly wash a wound out making the last wash a normal saline wash can help maintain the right osmolality but this is not essential

Chapter 7 The Basic Laboratory

The basics of a diagnosis can generally be reached by a careful history and physical examination. Modern medicine relies heavily on laboratory investigations. In a survival situation these will not be available. However there are some simple laboratory tests which can be performed with very little equipment or chemicals. The problem is that even basic tests require some equipment ranging from simple test strips to a microscope and a few chemicals. Obviously what you are preparing for will dictate what tests you may want to be able to perform.

Urine Testing: Urine is easily tested with multi-function dip stix. These can test for the presence of protein, glucose, ketones, nitrates, red blood cells, and white blood cells. The test strip is dipped in a specimen of clean catch urine (i.e. urination begins in the toilet, stop, then start again into the specimen container, stop, and continue into the toilet) and panels containing the test reagents change colour depending on the presence and concentrations of the substance being tested for. The colour changes are compared to a table supplied with the strips. The strips can be used to diagnose urinary infections, toxaemia in pregnancy, dehydration, diabetes (outside pregnancy), and renal stones/colic.

Contents

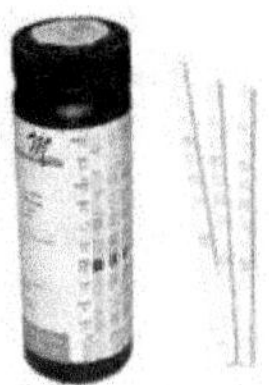

These urinalysis reagent strips test for the following:

- Leukocytes
- Nitrite
- Urobilinogen
- Bilirubin
- Ketones
- Protein
- PH
- Specific gravity
- Glucose
- Blood

Cost is approximately US$ 40 per 100 strips.

The following is a quote on analysing urine from a book to be published on the practice of medicine under relatively primitive conditions.

****

From: Roberts, S. D.; A Guide to the Practice of Medicine Under Austere Conditions (Revised Ed.), to be published.

Urinalysis

Of the various bodily fluids urine is the most easily obtained. It is possible to perform a number of tests on urine with little or no equipment. Visual and olfactory

Contents

examination of a urine sample alone can provide considerable information. Urine which is pink, red, or red-orange may contain blood although it is important to remember that these colors may also be seen in those who have eaten certain foods such as beets, blackberries, or rhubarb. Urine which is green or blue-green, or which takes on these hues on standing may indicate diseases of the liver or gall bladder.

Bright yellow or yellow-orange urine is indicative of kidney dysfunction (if there is no reason for the urine to be concentrated and if the colour is maintained for several days). Cloudy urine may result from abnormally high levels of phosphates or carbonates in the urine, and may be a precursor of kidney stones. Cloudy urine may also indicate the presence of an infection particularly if the fresh urine has an odour of ammonia or other disagreeable odour (note that urine will develop an ammonia odour on standing).

It is possible to approximately localize an infection that is producing cloudy urine by using the three-glass test. This test requires three clean containers (glasses) of which at least one (the second used) will need a capacity of at least 500 ml. In this test, the first 5 ml is voided into the first container, the second container is used until the patient is almost done, and then the third container is used to collect the last 5 ml. If the urine in the first container is the cloudiest, with decreasing cloudiness in the remaining containers, a urethral infection is the most likely cause. If the urine in the first container is less cloudy than either of the following two, a kidney, bladder, or prostate infection is indicated as the cause while if the urine in the third container is

the cloudiest the prostate is the likely site of the infection.

The odour of maple syrup associated with fresh urine is, of course, the classic sign of maple syrup urine disease. The urine may also have characteristic odors which are associated with other genetic disorders: the `mousy' odor associated with phenylketonuria for instance; the presence of glucose in urine has long been recognized as an indication of diabetes and its detection has been assigned a high degree of importance by the general public. While its presence was at one time detected by taste a more aesthetically acceptable method (which is also less likely to transmit infection) is to heat the urine and observe the odor. If the scent of burning sugar or caramel is detected there is an excessive amount of sugar present.

Proteins, or carbonates and phosphates in urine may be detected by filling a test tube three-fourths full of urine and boiling the upper portion. Any cloudiness produced by this may arise from either the presence of carbonates and phosphates (which may be normal) or from the presence of proteins. These two causes may be differentiated by adding a small amount of acetic acid (3-5 drops of 10% acetic acid) to the tube: if the cloudiness vanishes carbonates and phosphates were the cause; if the cloudiness persists or becomes apparent only after the acid is added, proteins are present.

The iodine ring test is a simple test which can detect the presence of bile in the urine before colour changes or jaundice make its presence obvious. In this test the appearance of a green ring after layering a 10% alcoholic iodine solution over the urine in a test tube indicates the presence of bile.

■■■

Blood Counts:

Contents

There is no easy way to do blood counts without some basic equipment. You need a microscope and a graded slide. A graded slide is a microscope slide which has very small squares etched onto its surface. Using a standardized technique a smear of blood is placed on the slide. Now using the microscope the number of different types of blood cells in a square on the slide is counted, this is then repeated several times and then averaged. This technique will give you:

- White Cell count
- White Cell differential
- Red Cell count
- Platelet count

This graded slide is called a hemacytometer and can be found frequently on auction sites such as e-Bay at a price of $15-$50 USD. The hemacytometer frequently comes as a kit with two graduated pipettes, the hemacytometer itself, the cover slip, and hopefully a set of instructions for that particular hemacytometer. The basic procedure is to dilute the sample to a given ratio and place that sample on the tiny grid etched into the glass of the hemacytometer. A cover slip is a precise set distance from the bottom of the slide creating a known volume for each of the squares. The sample and the hemacytometer are then viewed through the microscope. The idea is to count how many cells appear in the squares. Several squares are counted and taken into account to average out the number.

For example: You dilute the sample of blood to a 1:20 with a 1% acetic acid solution (diluted white vinegar can possibly be used in place of the glacial acetic acid). You then place it under the microscope and count eight 1 square mm area, and get a total number of 300 white cells. Then use the formula:

Cells counted X dilution X 10 Number of 1 sq. mm areas counted

-or-

300 X 20 X 10

8

= 7,500 white cells per cc of blood.

Red blood cell counts can also be done in this manner, with slightly different preparation and procedure although a hematocrit (percentage of red blood cells in whole blood) is more commonly used for diagnosis.

Contents

The hematocrit test consists essentially of drawing a blood sample, adding a small amount of anticoagulant to prevent clotting (such as sodium citrate or heparin), and placing a sample in a very tiny glass tube called a capillary tube. The capillary tube end is sealed with a clay-like substance, centrifuged for 5 minutes at 2000 rpm. The packed red blood cell volume is determined by comparison with a standard scale on a micro hematocrit reader.

NOTE: The picture below is for illustration purposes only. DO NOT attempt to use it as the hematocrit scale!

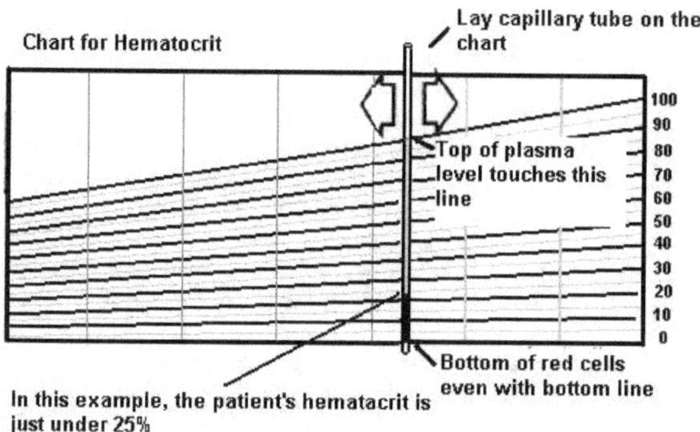

Blood Grouping:

Patient Blood Type	Can Receive:							
	O-	O+	B-	B+	A-	A+	AB-	AB+
AB+								
AB-								
A+								
A-								
B+								
B-								
O+								
O-								

There are four basic blood types: A, B, AB, and O. There is also an additional subgroup of each type of blood, Rh+ or Rh-. Some of these blood groups are compatible with one another some are not.

Contents

This chart shows the

patients blood type on the vertical axis on the left, and the donor's blood type across the top. Note that O- blood type can be given to any patient, and that a

patient with AB+ blood type can receive blood from anyone. There are other further subdivisions of

blood which can make a whole-blood transfusion not as simple as the chart above, but it's a starting point. The simplest thing to do is have your group or expedition blood typed prior to your expedition or a disaster. However, provided you have several basic chemicals a cross match is a simple test. If you are unable or unwilling to have this done (usually the Red Cross will give you a donor card with that information on it when you donate blood) there is another method that is nearly as simple. For economic reasons usually ABO and Rh has been done using liquid anti-A, anti-B, and anti-D (anti-D tests Rh +/-) sera on slides mixed with drops of blood. Then the drops were observed to see which agglutinated or "clumped together". There is a method to dry the anti-A, anti-B, and anti-D sera and put the whole test on a pre-made card commonly called an "Eldon Card." These cards are about $6-$10 USD, and are becoming more common due to a diet that dictates your food choices based on blood type. The cards have a shelf life of roughly three years when stored in the refrigerator. ABO typing with sera is well-described in any basic laboratory medicine textbook.

Cross matching:

Just having compatible ABO/Rh is not enough to assure a safe blood transfusion. To be certain that a transfusion will be safe a direct compatibility or "cross match" test is performed. There are several ways to perform a cross match. A saline cross match and an albumin cross match are two of them. The albumen cross match consists of a drop of 30% bovine albumin added to a saline cross match. It requires bovine - cow- albumin which may not be available in austere conditions. Under ideal conditions both types of cross match are performed, and more.

Saline Cross match Method:

Contents

1. Take a few drops of the donor blood to be cross matched and place it into a tube full of saline (0.9%).
2. Spin with a centrifuge.
3. You will be left with a small deposit of washed red cells in the bottom of the tube. Pipette (draw) off the saline to leave a deposit of nearly dry washed red cells.
4. Add fresh saline solution to the cells in the bottom of the tube. You will add saline until there is approximately twenty times as much saline as red cells. Don't make the suspension too weak.
5. Separate the cells from the serum of the patient's blood by placing a sample in a tube and spinning it with a centrifuge. The cells will once again be in the bottom of the tube with the serum on top.
6. Place two drops of the suspension in a fresh, clean, sterile tube and add two drops of the patient's serum.
7. Mix and keep at body temperature for two hours.
8. Observe sample with a microscope. If the cells are clumping and sticking together this is agglutination, and the donor's blood should not be given. Sometimes cells will be stacked into neat rolls like stacks of coins. This is different from agglutination. This is called "rouleaux" and it is safe to give the donor's blood. Usually the rouleaux is easy to differentiate from agglutination but sometimes it is not. If not certain, do not give the donor's blood to the patient.

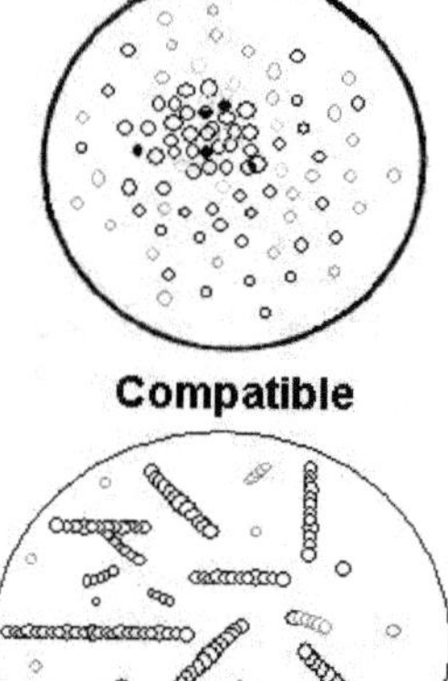

Compatible

Compatible: Rouleaux

Contents

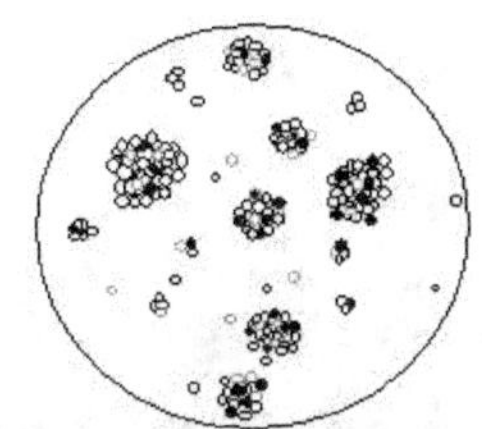

Incompatible: Agglutination

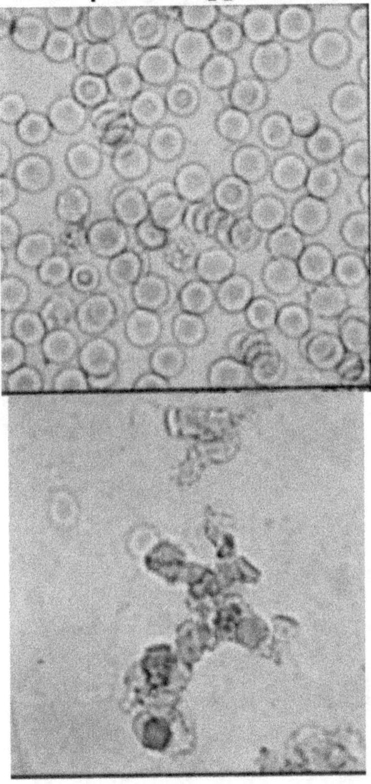

Contents

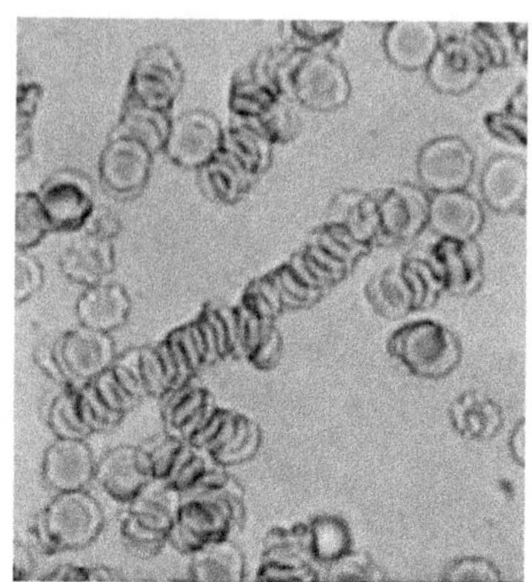

Gram Staining:

This is a technique for approximate identification of bacteria in urine, pus, sputum, cerebral spinal fluid (CSF), and from bacterial cultures. Although not highly accurate in species identification combined with knowledge of the clinical situation it enables a good guess to be made for the appropriate antibiotic. It requires a microscope and also several chemical solutions.

The Gram stain is the most widely used staining procedure in bacteriology. It is called a differential stain since it differentiates between gram-positive and gram-negative bacteria. Bacteria that stain purple with the Gram staining procedure are called gram- positive; those that stain pink are said to be gram-negative. Gram-positive and gram- negative bacteria stain differently because of differences in the structure of their cell walls.

The gram staining procedure involves four basic steps:

1. The bacteria are first stained with the basic dye crystal violet. Both gram-positive and gram-negative bacteria become directly stained and appear purple after this step.
2. The bacteria are then treated with an iodine solution. This allows the stain to be retained better. Both gram-positive and gram-negative bacteria remain purple after this step.
3. Decolouriser is then added. This is the differential step. Gram-positive bacteria retain the crystal violet-iodine complex while gram-negative are decolorized.
4. Finally, the counterstain safranine is applied. Since the gram-positive bacteria are already stained purple they are not affected by the counterstain. Gram-negative bacteria that are now colourless become directly stained by the safranine. Thus, gram- positive appear purple and gram-negative appear pink.

It is important to note that gram-positivity (the ability to retain the purple crystal violet-iodine complex) is not an all-or-nothing phenomenon but a matter of degree.

Contents

There are several factors that could result in a gram-positive organism staining gram- negatively:

1. The method and techniques used. Overheating during heat fixation, over decolourisation with alcohol, and even too much washing with water between steps may result in gram-positive bacteria losing the crystal violet-iodine complex.
2. The age of the culture. Cultures more than 24 hours old may lose their ability to retain the crystal violet-iodine complex.
3. The organism itself. Some gram-positive bacteria are more able to retain the crystal violet-iodine complex than others.

Therefore, one must use very precise techniques in gram staining and interpret the results with discretion.

Procedure

1. Heat-fix a smear of a mixture of the bacterium as follows:
    1. Using the dropper bottle of distilled water place a small drop of water on a clean slide by touching the dropper to the slide.
    2. Ideally, should this sample be from a wound it would be cultured on an agar plate, and then a sample colony of cells would be transferred to the slide with a sterilized wire loop. Failing that, take a small sample from the exudates of the wound directly with the sterilized wire loop.
    3. Using the loop spread the mixture over the entire slide to form a thin film.
    4. Allow this thin suspension to completely air dry.
    5. Pass the slide (film-side up) through the flame of the Bunsen burner 3 or 4 times to heat-fix the sample. Never allow any portion of the slide to become hot to the touch.
2. Flood the slide with crystal violet (solution of 0.3% crystal violet in 0.8% ammonium oxalate) and let stand for one minute and then gently wash off with water. Shake off the excess water but do not blot dry between steps.
3. Stain with iodine solution (0.33% iodine + 0.66% potassium iodide in water) for one minute then gently wash with water.
4. Decolorize by adding gram decolouriser (Ethanol:acetone solution 1:1) drop by drop until the purple stops flowing then wash immediately with water.
5. Stain with safranine (0.25% safranine, aqueous solution) for one minute then wash with water.
6. Blot or air dry, and observe using oil immersion lens on your microscope at 1000x magnification.

You may call the cells that you see either gram-positive or gram-negative.

Further classify bacteria by their shape and pattern.

Cocci (singular: Coccus) are generally spherical though with some variation from this theme (i.e., elongation or flattening on one side).

Contents

1. Diplococci: Cocci that remain in pairs after they divide
2. Streptococci: Cocci that fail to separate after they divide but instead remain in chains of cells.
3. Tetrad: Cocci that fail to separate after they divide but instead remain in groups of four forming squares.
4. Sarcinae: Cocci that fail to separate after they divide but instead remain in groups of eight forming cubes.
5. Staphylococci: Cocci that fail to separate after they divide but instead remain in amorphous sheets or clumps.

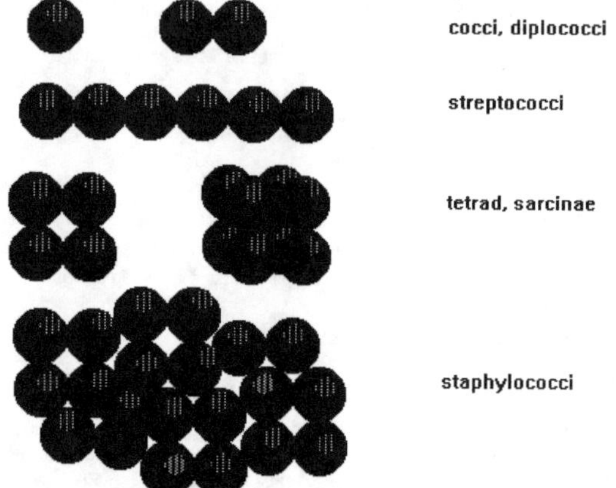

Bacilli (singular: Bacillus) are rods or variations on rod-shaped bacteria: tapered rod, staff, cigar, oval, or curve shaped. Basically, *bacilli* are longer than they are wide and lack extreme curvature.

1. Diplobacilli: Paired rods that remain in pairs after they divide.
2. Streptobacilli: Rods that fail to separate after they divide but instead remain in chains of cells.
3. Coccobacilli: A short rod that nearly looks like cocci.

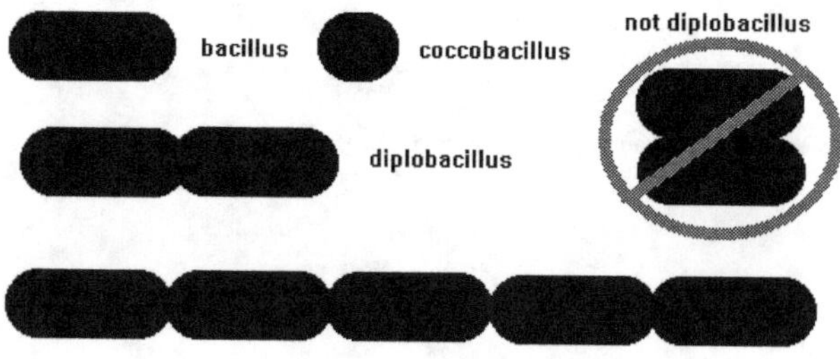

Additional bacterial shapes include:

Contents

Adding the shape and arrangement of the bacteria to the gram-negative or positive status can help you to select the proper antibiotic. Many further tests must be done to isolate the actual specific bacterial organism. Knowing the gram status and general morphology (shape and pattern) can aid in eliminating possible antibiotic treatments. Most often clinical experience and history is the best indicator of treatment regimen.

Growing Bacteria: Most bacteria can be grown on simple agar plates. There are some which are difficult to grow (e.g. the bacteria causing TB), but the majority will grow. A sample of body fluid – urine, pus, sputum, etc. is spread on an agar plate using a sterilised (by direct heating in a flame) piece of wire in a narrow zigzag pattern. The plates are then cultured at temperatures in the high 30s Celsius. The colonies which grow can then be examined using the above techniques.

Agar plates can be made using the following techniques:

The agar should be placed into shallow dishes with a lid – Petri dishes (100 mm by 15 mm) are what are traditionally used but you can improvise

Dissolve a vegetable stock cube and a gelling agent, usually 15 grams (1/2 oz) of agar, or one pack of all propose gelatine, or one jelly desert mix, in 1/2 cup (125 ml) of distilled boiling water. Make sure the gelling agent contains agar, carrageen, or guar gum.

To resterilize the dishes and lids place them in boiling distilled water. Leave them in the water to cool.

Pour the agar into a shallow Petri dish. It will form a jelly in each dish. Put the lid on and leave until the jelly is set. Store the dishes upside-down until you need them. This will stop water condensation from falling on the jelly.

A suitable reference would be: Benson, Harold J; Microbiological Applications: A Laboratory Manual in General Microbiology Short Version (Paperback, 2001)

Pregnancy Tests:

The ability to accurately diagnose pregnancy may be important both for psychological reasons and for practical reasons. Currently available pregnancy test kits will test urine for the presence of the hormone Human chorionic gonadotrophin (HCG). They require only a small amount of urine and are accurate from 10-14 days from conception. The tests available in common grocery stores are nearly as sensitive as a laboratory test, in fact many Emergency Departments rely on this type for their rapid tests. These tests are inexpensive and widely available. Follow directions included with packaging.

Blood Glucose test strips:

Also known as "BM stix," after a common brand. These can be used to diagnose diabetes (in a survival situation); both general and during pregnancy, also it can detect low or high blood sugars in other severe illnesses. A finger or toe is pricked and a drop of capillary blood is collected onto a test strip. It's allowed to sit for 30 seconds and then wiped off. After a further 90 seconds the colour of the test strip is compared to a control chart to give a blood glucose level reading. Test strips which do not rely on an electronic reader are becoming increasingly rare. An electronic glucometer can be had initially for a small investment, but as a general rule the most inexpensive meters require the most expensive consumable strips. Though more accurate, for truly austere and disaster care, weigh their cost, necessary reliance upon batteries, and consumable test strips. They are available at nearly every pharmacy.

Other infectious disease test kits are manufactured. However, their availability is not common. Many are not approved by the US Food and Drug Administration and are, therefore, not for sale in the US. Tests for Chlamydia, Syphilis, Malaria, H. pylori, and mononucleosis fall into these categories. For residents of other countries some research will need to be performed to find if these tests are available in your country.

Chapter 8 Botanical and Herbal Medicine

(Note. The following is an introduction to Herbal and Botanical Medicine with a special orientation to preparedness and survival situations. It is written by an author with an interest in herbalism and preparedness. It is offered in good faith. The scientific evidence supporting some of the botanical preparations mentioned here is variable – from strong evidence to anecdote. The "bible" on scientific herbalism is "Medical Botany: Plants Affecting Human Health" by Lewis and Lewis, Published by Wiley 2003. This book deals in-depth with the evidence base for botanical medicine and cannot be recommended highly enough. It is not "how-to" book but a scientific treatise on the subject.

We strongly recommend you consult a reputable herbal identification and medicine text prior to undertaking any treatments discussed here. Also note that this section has a slight North American bias due the chapter writer's location, but much can be generalised)

Contents

Many of the present day pharmaceuticals were derived from botanicals or herbs. They can be very complimentary to conventional medications and have a valid track record of treating, easing, and resolving many diseases. While some may have not therapeutic effect at all the reason most have been used consistently for centuries by various cultures is because they work – the efficacy may vary, but they do work to some degree or another. The incidence of serious side effects with herbs and botanicals appears to be low although like anything taken excessively or misused can result in serious adverse effects. There is also a small potential for interactions with conventional medication, and botanical medicines should be prescribed with the full knowledge of other medications the patient is taking.

Botanicals and herbs work in several complimentary ways. Firstly they can treat illness and disease directly as with most medications. Many, however, work at building the body's natural defences and affect the more root cause of disease. Most botanicals/herbs work slowly with the body and do their work for the most part gently, unobtrusively, and supportively.

In order to utilise botanicals/herbs in a survival situation you need to plan ahead. Botanicals/herbs are not just another "prep" item to add to your list - planning ahead in this case most certainly will involve a little more work and time than just buying what you think you need and storing it away.

Botanical/herb therapies and treatments seem to lend themselves more to a "Bug In" situation rather than a "Bug Out" scenario mostly because it would be difficult to have the added weight of a couple of quarts of tincture in your pack and in a long term lack of conventional medical facilities in order to continue to have the botanicals and herbs available you really need to grow them or know where to gather them in your local area.

We strongly suggest you get at least one really good medicinal herb identification

book. These are available for most countries and areas. A useful series of books in the US are the Peterson Field Guides. The older editions were two books; one for the Eastern U.S. and one for the Western U.S. There are now newer editions: A Field Guide to Medicinal Plants and Herbs of Eastern and Central North America by S. Foster and James Duke and A Field Guide to Western Medicinal Plants and Herbs by

S. Foster. There many other excellent guides available some very localised to specific areas.

There are two excellent books focusing on the pharmacology of botanical medicines. In addition to these textbook styles there are many other excellent books on herbal medicine although there is some significant variation in how strong the science behind the books are. Don't buy any book blindly, get your local library to special order books for you to read, and then decide if that one would be of use to you.

Contents

The next step is becoming familiar with what is growing wild in your local area. It can be as simple as taking Sunday afternoon nature walks with the family starting in mid to late spring. Do this again in early summer - same areas as before. As you identify herbs/botanicals make a mental or even paper map of these locations. Do your walk again in late summer/early fall and check locations because many herbs and plants need to be harvested before flowering, or after flowering, or after having died down.

If you don't have a location map you may not be able to find that clump of purple coneflower (Echinacea) when it has no leaves and no purple flower.

Preparation of fresh botanicals and herbs for storage

Leaves:

Harvested botanical and herb leaves are traditionally dried to concentrate the medicinal properties. If you have a gas stove with a pilot light in the oven just spread the leaves 1 layer thick on cookie sheets and put in the oven. The heat from the pilot light will dry the leaves perfectly in a day or so. Check the progress and remove leaves from the oven when they crumble between your fingers. You can also use a food dehydrator with the thermostat set between 250-275 degrees F. Overnight is usually enough.

For fat, thick, juicy type leaves such as mullein or comfrey tie the leaves in small bunches (about 4-6) and hang from a line or rack in a dark warm room.

Another option is to make drying screens out of 1 x 2s - any size you like - covered with old plastic screen material, attach lines to the corners, and attach those lines to hooks in the ceiling of a dark, warm room. You can use these same screens to air dry outside but not in direct sunshine. Slow and gentle are the bywords for drying herbs. High humidity will slow down the process.

Store your dried leaves in quart-sized Zip-lock bags with air in the bags or tightly capped jars in a dark place. You do not want to crush the dried leaves at this stage. Be sure and clearly label as to the herb and year harvested. Most dried herb/botanical

leaves will maintain their potency for 2 years this way.

Roots/bark/twigs:

Roots, bark, and twigs are traditionally dried. You should chop the fresh root, bark, or twigs BEFORE drying. A dried whole root or twig resembles a wrinkled railroad spike and is just as hard; they can be impossible to chop or crush if dried whole.

Contents

Wash the root clean of dirt with cool running water, chop, and dry using the same techniques as for leaves. It takes twice as long to dry roots and twigs. There should be NO moisture in the dried root/twig/ bark or it will mould and be useless. I usually try to split open a piece of root/twig with a sharp knife - if it cuts open easily it's not dry enough yet.

Flowers:

Harvested flowers are traditionally dried. Just spread the flower heads out and dry using the same as the leaf drying techniques. Store the same as leaves.

Whole herb:

Occasionally the whole plant may be used in formulas. In that case just

hang the whole plant upside down in a dark, warm room until the main stem snaps.

Medicinal Botanical preparation methods:

Having gathered your dried herbs and botanicals, what do you do with them to be able to best use their medicinal components? Keep in mind that botanical and herbal preparations are not made and used with precise measurements or dosages. Herbs and botanicals vary greatly in the potency of their medicinal components due to weather, growing conditions, and soil conditions. The traditional measurements/dosages are used primarily based on the minimum found to be effective. There are a few herbs/botanicals which are toxic or can cause negative reactions due to an overdose.

There is a degree of trial and error with dosing. You should initially be conservative in your initial dosages.

Water infusions/tea:

Medicinal teas are a time-honoured, traditional usage of herbs and botanicals. It is an easy way to treat children or someone who is very ill. A preferred method is to get one of those silvery tea balls, stuff it full of crushed, not powdered, dried herb, put it in a cup, pour boiling water into the cup, let sit (steep) covered if possible, for about 10 minutes. Add some honey if sweetener is needed and sip away. The dosage varies

with the herb, but a cup 3-4 times a day is reasonably standard.

Medicinal teas must be very strong in order to be potent. They frequently taste very bad. The exception to this would be using a very mild herbal tea for infants and children - smaller body mass and weight so teas need to be less strong and ,therefore, more palatable for them.

Contents

If the tea you want to use needs to be used throughout the day make up a quart jar full using 1 tea ball of herb per cup of water, strain after steeping if using loose herbs, and it's ready for use when needed for the day. It will keep safely 24 hours without refrigeration, 2-3 days with refrigeration.

Oil infusion:

Oil infusions are handy for skin infections, itchy, dry skin, burns, and as ear drops.

Take dried herbs, crush (not powder) put enough in a glass

baking pan to cover the bottom thinly, and cover the herbs with olive oil. Olive oil will not go rancid so you can make this ahead of time and store on the shelf. Stir the oil and herbs to make sure all herbs are coated with oil, then cover with more oil to at least 1/2 inch. If you have a gas stove with an oven pilot light just leave the pan of herbs and oil in the oven overnight. Alternatively, set the pan of herbs and oil in the sun for about 2 weeks with some sort of lightweight fabric covering it to protect from bugs. Strain the oil out through a cloth with a tight weave, bottle it, and use as needed topically.

Salve:

Herbal/botanical salves are just an oil infusion hardened with beeswax. You need lots of the oil infusion. Put the oil infusion in a glass or stainless steel cooking pot and heat gently. Add chopped/shaved beeswax to the warmed oil; usually 2oz beeswax per cup of oil. When the beeswax is melted place a few drops on a saucer, let cool, and touch it. It is too soft add more beeswax to the pot; if too hard add a bit more oil to the pot. The perfect salve should stay hard for a few seconds as you gently press your finger on it then suddenly soften from your body heat. Pour into appropriate containers for use as needed.

Decoction:

Decoctions are herbs/botanicals prepared in boiling water used primarily for compresses and syrups. If you have NO taste buds it can be drunk! Use approximately a heaping palmful of dried, crushed (not powdered) herb per pint of water. Boil together for about 15 minutes, cool, strain and add sufficient water to bring the volume back to a pint. For compresses just soak a sterile dressing in the liquid and apply to the body. To make a syrup add sufficient honey to thicken and make

palatable. Good treatment for sore throats.

Steams:

Contents

Steams utilise the inhalation route. Put 1-2 hands full of dried, crushed (not powdered) herb or fresh (best if available as whole leaf) into a large pot filled with water. Stew or spaghetti pots are good but not aluminium. Bring the water to a boil with the herbs in the water, place pot on a table, cover the head and pot with a towel, hang head over the pot, and breathe deep. Take sensible precautions to avoid burns from the pot and/or water and steam. When no steam is rising, reheat to boiling, and repeat treatment. When the herbs no longer have a scent in the stream you can add more and continue the treatment until desired relief is achieved.

Tinctures:

Tinctures are an alcohol-based extraction that is medicinally the most potent herbal

treatment. When you dry herbs/botanicals the medicinal components are concentrated with the removal of the water. Soaking (tincturing) the dried herb/botanical in alcohol extracts those concentrated medicinal components and makes them available. An additional bonus is that alcohol-based tinctures are medicinally potent for years if stored in dark bottles or jars. We tincture most of our herbs and botanicals so they are immediately available for use, and we can be confident they are potent in an acute situation. We also keep dried herbs available for infant/child usage as teas, and also particular dried herbs available for poultices, and compress, and topical usage.

To prepare the tincture you need quart canning jars with lids, dried herbs/botanicals, and at least 90 proof Vodka. Everclear is excellent to use also and in a pinch you could use another grain-based product. You want the alcohol to become saturated with the medicinal components of the herb/botanical, and other alcohol liquors/whiskey have components already saturating the alcohol so it probably won't be as medicinally potent, but it would still have more potency that other preparation methods. Fill the quart jar about 1/3 full of dried herb/botanical, chopped root, or crushed (not powdered) leaf, fill the jar to the "shoulder" with vodka/Everclear, secure the lid, shake, and put in a dark cool place. Every 2nd or 3rd day give it a shake. In 10-14 days strain the liquid into dark bottles or jars, cap tightly, and label.

The commonly accepted tincture dosage is 1-2 eye droppers full, 1 dropper full equals approximately 1/2 teaspoon. Place half to one teaspoon of tincture in a glass of water and drink. Alternatively, you can use the dropper to place the tincture in gelatine capsules. You can also use tinctures to make a nasal spray for sinus congestion/infection. Buy some of those empty 1 oz (30 ml) nasal spray bottles at the drug store, put 8-10 DROPS of tincture in the bottle, fill the bottle with distilled water, and use as often as needed, 1-2 sprays per nostril.

Capsules:

An easy reliable preparation is herbal/botanical capsules. You can buy empty gelatine capsules in health food stores by the capsule or by the bag of 1000. Just pop the capsule apart, fill the larger section with finely crushed (powdered) dried herb, put

back together, and take with water.

Contents

Poultice:

A poultice is warm, mashed, fresh, or finely crushed dried herb applied directly to the skin to relieve inflammation, bites, eruptions, boils, and abscesses. Depending on the size of the area to be treated put enough herbs in a glass dish/pot, cover with enough olive oil, or water, or decoction of the same herb to thoroughly saturate the herb, heat gently until a comfortable temperature to the skin, apply directly to the area to be treated covering it completely, and then cover with a sterile bandage. Repeat the treatment as needed.

Bolus/Suppository:

These are made using vegetable glycerine or cocoa butter mixed with a dried powdered herb to the consistency of bread dough. You may have to add some wheat flour to get this consistency. Shape the dough into a suppository shape and chill to set the form. When needed for use let warm a bit on the counter then insert appropriately. This method allows the herb to be in direct contact with the area needing treatment.

Syrup:

To about a pint of decoction you add enough honey and/or eatable glycerine to thicken slightly. Licorice or wild cherry bark are commonly added as flavouring. Especially good for children to treat coughs, congestions, and sore throat as it will coat these areas slightly ,and keep the medicinal components in direct contact with the tissues.

Specific Herbs and Botanicals

We have tried to refine a list of herbs/botanicals, both wildcrafted and home grown, that would be most useful in treating the most common illnesses or diseases that may manifest in a survival situation. From the reading you have been doing in your newly acquired herb information books you now realize the vast amount of information and herbs available for use. Just use this list as a starting point to adjust and personalize according to your needs and medical situations.

Wildcrafting:

The following 7 herbs and botanicals grow almost universally all over the U.S. and many more widely. Some are considered weeds.

Contents

1. Burdock (Arctium lappa): Harvest 1st year roots in the fall. Tincture or water infusion. Used internally Burdock will help with arthritis. Used as a poultice or compress Burdock will reduce swelling around joints. It has a blood cleanser effect (detoxifier) and is nutritive to the liver; also mildly diuretic.
2. Dandelion (Taraxacum officinale): Harvest 2nd year roots in the spring or fall; young leaves in the spring for fresh eating. Tincture, water infusion, syrup. Dandelion is a potent diuretic used internally as a tincture or water infusion. The root has been used for centuries to treat jaundice as it has a powerful alterative effect on the liver. Dandelion syrup is a good treatment for tonsillitis discomfort.
3. Echinacea (Echinacea angustifolia): Harvest 2nd and 3rd year roots in early winter after the plant has totally died back (see, you do need your map!). Echinacea purpurea: Harvest flower heads with seeds before petals drop in late summer. Tincture, water infusion, oil infusion, decoction, poultice, compress, bolus, syrup, capsule. Using these two varieties together gives increases the potency of your treatments. Used internally Echinacea has been found to stimulate the immune response system. For strengthening the immune system dosage suggested is a dropper full (1/2 tsp) daily for a 10-day course, no herb for 7 days, then repeat the 10-day course, etc. Used on this basis it is a flu and cold preventive.

It is also considered to have antiinflammatory and antimicrobial properties. This herb is a whole pharmacy within itself. An absolute must have in your survival stash. If you can only have one herb in your survival pharmacy make it Echinacea. One option now is to purchase 1# of cut and sifted Echinacea angustifolia root (currently $23/lb), tincture half of it right now, and save half for future decoctions and poultices. This will give you some time to gather your own root, and the tincture will be medicinally potent for at least 10 years.

Echinacea root tincture has activity against influenza, herpes, and other viruses which includes virus which cause the common colds. Echinacea decoction or tincture can be used effectively to treat gingivitis. Just soak a cotton ball or swab in the decoction and apply directly to the gums twice daily until the disease is resolved. Echinacea has a numbing effect on the tissues. There is anecdotal evidence Echinacea may be an effective treatment for athlete's foot, bladder infections, bursitis/tendinitis, Lyme disease, pneumonia, sinusitis, tonsillitis, viral infections, and yeast infections used

both internally and externally.

1. Mullein (Verbascum thapsus): Harvest leaves before flowering taking no more than 1/3 of the total. Tincture, decoction, water infusion, syrup. Mullein is an excellent treatment for respiratory complaints. It has expectorant action, soothes the throat, has bactericidal activity, and helps stop muscle spasms that trigger coughs.

Mullein provides excellent relief and protection against air-born allergens. It seems to give mucous membranes a protective coating that allergens cannot penetrate. A 1 tsp dose protects against allergy symptoms for 4-5 hours with no negative side effects.

Mullein has been stated to have narcotic properties without being habit forming or

poisonous. It is said to be a strong painkiller and helps to induce sleep. We have not experienced these effects using mullein.

Contents

1. Plantin (Plantago major): Harvest leaves before seeds form in early summer. Fresh, poultice, salve. Plantain is primarily a proven healer of injured skin cells, hence the topical usage.

A salve or compress of plantain applied appropriately is known to reduce hemorrhoid swelling and pain. Fresh leaf crushed and tubbed on insect bites relieves pain and swelling. The New England Journal of Medicine carried a study reporting that poultices made from plantain leaves can help control the itching of poison ivy exposures, it is also good for poison oak also.

1. Red Clover (Trifolium pratense): Harvest flower heads in early summer. Tincture, water infusion, salve, syrup. Red clover tea or tincture taken daily is of great benefit in relieving symptoms of menopause as it is estrogenic. It is also of benefit in relieving menstrual cramps by taking daily during the menstrual time.

Red clover salve is real useful in treating burns. It is very useful for treating children because of its mild sedative effect and excellent for coughs, wheezing, and bronchitis.

1. Willow (Salix, any variety)

If you are allergic to aspirin do not use willow in any form as it contains salicin which is converted to salicylic acid

Harvest bark and twigs in the fall. Tincture, water infusion, decoction, compress, poultice, capsule.

If you are taking an aspirin a day for heart attack risk/angina prevention switching to 1 tsp of willow bark made into 1 cup of tea daily provides the same protection. That tea dosage is equivalent to approximately an 81 mg aspirin. For larger dosage amounts, tincture is most useful keeping in mind the tincture will take about 1 hour to reduce pain. Placing drops of tincture directly on a corn, bunion, or wart daily for 5-7 days usually removes the corn, bunion, or wart. Pain relief lasts up to 7 or 8 hours.

Home-grown/Cultivated Herbs and Botanicals

These next herbs are fairly easy to grow in a home garden as they usually do not grow in the wild. You need to start growing these plants now to have them established in case you really might need them.

1. Aloe (Aloe vera): Use fresh leaves as needed; cut a leaf close to the bottom of the plant, split it open, and use the gel inside topically on burns, minor cuts, and even radiation burns. Antibacterial, wound healing accelerator, antiinflammatory.

Most commonly found in a kitchen window in a pot, handy for instant use. You can buy potted aloe plants at grocery stores, or nurseries, or get your neighbor to give you one. They live a long time and set new plants from shoots off the roots. You can separate these shoots from the roots of the mother plant and pot separately at 1-2" tall. They thrive best in light with well-drained soil, and do not require frequent watering.

1. Catnip (Nepeta cataria): Harvest whole flowering tops and leaves. Dry for water infusions, tincture.

Contents

An excellent muscle relaxer/muscle pain killer including menstrual cramps: outstanding treatment for colic, restlessness, and pain reliever for small children; commonly called nature's "Alka Seltzer" for its stomach settling properties.

Commonly grown from seed sown in the fall but can be grown from root divisions from a parent plant in the spring. Space roots/seeds about 2' apart as catnip can get quite large - up to 4'; does well in full or partial sun. We have never been able to germinate the seed, so purchase starts from the local nursery. The plant will self-seed if you leave some flowers on.

1. Comfrey (Symphytum officinale): Harvest leaves before flowering throughout the growing season. You can harvest 2-3 times from the same plant remembering to take no more than 1/3 the total leaves. Dry or use fresh for poultices, water infusions, oil infusion, salve, compress, and decoction.

Comfrey is right up there with Echinacea as a must have herb. Comfrey has a long history of use for treating sores, i.e. diabetic ulcers, indolent ulcers, and other wounds; contains a compound that promotes new cell growth. Apply comfrey as a compress, poultice, decoction soak/wash, or salve to sores or wounds daily until resolved; will also relieve swelling, and inflammation, and pain. Comfrey makes a wonderful water infusion that is extremely gentle yet powerful treatment for stomach, and bowel discomforts.

Comfrey is grown from root pieces. Just plant in the spring and stand back. It spreads via root extensions, needs moderate water, and partial sun.

1. Dill (Any variety): Harvest the leaves when the plant is established in the garden, about 1' tall, again, no more than 1/3 leaves per harvest; harvest seed when ripe usually mid summer depending on weather. Use fresh or dried as water infusion,

tincture.

Dill is regularly used to dispel flatulence, increase mother's milk, and treat/prevent congestion of breasts during nursing. Drink as a water infusion several cups a day or take a dropperful of tincture daily.

Dill is easy to grow from seed inside or out; likes partial sun but warmth; will self- seed if you don't harvest all the flower heads for pickles and medicinal use.

1. Echinacea - If you cannot find enough Echinacea in the wild do grow it. It's easy to start from seed if you wait until air temperatures are 70 or above to plant. Does well in raised beds or regular flower beds; likes an alkaline soil, full sun, and moderate moisture. Refer to Wildcrafting section for preparations and uses.
2. Garlic (Allium sativum): Harvest bulb in late summer when the top has died back, cure (let air dry a few days outside) in the shade then store inside. Use fresh/cured bulbs or cloves of the bulb as water infusion, oil infusion, syrup, tincture.

Contents

Garlic is best known for it's antibiotic action, and for being a hypotensive agent (lowering blood pressure), and is effective in lowering cholesterol. It has been used medicinally almost 5000 years. Extracts made from the whole clove of garlic have consistently shown a broad-spectrum antibiotic range effective against both gram- negative, and gram-positive bacteria, and most major infectious bacteria in laboratory studies. How this translates into action inside the body is not entirely clear and needs more research.

Garlic taken internally as fresh in solid or as a juice may cause nausea and vomiting.

Garlic is easy to grow; just plant individual cloves about 1-2" deep, 6" apart in the fall for big bulbs or in the spring for medium sized.

1. Hawthorn (Crategnus oxyacantha): Harvest berries in the fall. Dry or tincture. Hawthorn has significant cardiac effects. It appears safe for long-term regular use, i.e. daily for years. It may be useful in congestive heart failure, arrhythmias, enlarged heart, and for symptomatic relief from cardiac symptoms.

Hawthorn is a tree; grows to 20-25 ' tall. We would suggest planting several if heart disease/problems run in your family. Be sure that the Hawthorn you are growing is the correct species for the medicinal properties.

1. Parsley (Petroselinum sativum): Harvest leaves throughout the growing season taking no more than 1/2 the total each time. In the fall cut the whole plant down to about an inch or 2 from the ground. Dry or use fresh. Tincture, water infusion, fresh and raw.

Do not use parsley during pregnancy as it can precipitate labour.

A supportive therapy in liver disease when jaundice is present. A mild water infusion is a good eye wash treatment for conjunctivitis and blepharitis. It is very good for urinary tract infections and as a diuretic. Has been used to dry up breast milk, which would be useful for weaning. A traditional breath freshener.

Parsley seed is notoriously a slow germinator sometimes taking 2-3 weeks to sprout. Plant barely 1/2" deep in lots of compost. After you cut back in the fall throw a cover over it, and in the spring remove the cover, water, and it likely will come back for

another season.

1. Poppy (Papavar somniferum):

Be aware of the local legal status of poppies, and be aware that illegal possession of opiates has harsh penalties. Also note that there are a number of different poppies and most bought from the plant shop are not Papavar somniferum)

Harvest resin when the seed pod is fully formed, green, and juicy looking; harvest seed when the seed pod has dried, brown, and hard. Tincture, water infusion.

Contents

When the fully formed seed pod is fat, juicy looking, and still green use a small sharp knife tip to make 3-4 shallow slits 2/3rds the way down the seed pod from the top to bottom direction, space the cuts evenly around the pod. The resin will slowly ooze out and begin to air harden, daily scrape off the semi hardened resin from the cuts and (wearing surgical gloves) shape the resin into a ball shape. Store in a glass container, cool and dark. Each day form the newly collected resin onto the ball. When the resin no longer oozes make 3-4 new cuts, spaced between the old ones evenly, and repeat the process. Three series of cuts per pod is sufficient. When the seed pod fully dries, and turns brown, and hard, and you can hear the seeds rattle when you gently shake the pod, pick the whole pod, and break open over wax paper or paper towel to harvest the seeds. Let a few pods remain on the stems and the plant will self-seed for the next year.

You can tincture the seeds or resin and also use the seeds for a severe pain relieving tea to use if the patient is conscious. A dropperful of the tincture might be used by inserting under the tongue of an unconscious patient.

Poppy seeds are usually planted outside when the ground is warm in the spring, partial to full sun, moderate water. Will self-seed if pods left intact on the stem.

1. Red Raspberry (Rubys idaeus): Harvest leaves throughout the growing season taking no more than 1/3 of the total until frost, then strip the canes. Dry. Most effective as a water infusion. This is a safe and useful herb in pregnancy. It may strengthen the uterine muscle, ease or prevent nausea, help prevent haemorrhage, reduce labour pain, helps reduce or prevent false labour, help decrease uterine swelling after delivery, and reduces post partum bleeding. It also gives good relief of vomiting in sick children and is a good remedy for diarrhoea in infants.

Red Raspberry grows as 6-8 foot canes from spreading roots. Likes partial sun. Plant 1 year roots. Will produce for years.

1. St Johns Wort (Hypercicum perforatum): Harvest leaves before flowering. Dry, Tincture, water infusion. Grows wild in many places but most states list it as a noxious weed and spray it every chance they get. You don't want sprayed leaves. Best bet is to surreptitiously dig up a few sprouts and transplant onto your property.

St. John's Wort has many medicinal properties but is currently best known as a proven antidepressant with absolutely no side effects.

NOTE: St John Worts is a monoamine oxidase inhibitor so the same food restrictions apply to St Johns Wort as to pharmaceutical MAOIs – wine, cheese, and other foods. Exercise caution

We feel it may be extremely important to have an antidepressant available during a long-term survival situation, one you can safely take, and still keep functioning well on a mental and physical level.

A couple of additional plants worthy of mention:

- 1. Foxglove (Digitalis pupurea)

Contents

Digitalis is a cardiac glycoside; it improves how the heart pumps when the cardiac muscle is failing, and it also slows the heart rate in a condition called atrial fibrillation which improves its efficiency. Foxglove has been used to treat these conditions for centuries; it has only been in the last 200 years that Digitalis was identified as the active ingredient.

Traditionally it was made into an infusion and drunk. An overdose of Foxglove can be fatal. Like any botanical medicine, in the absence of scientific testing of concentrations, there is degree of trial and error, however, you need to be aware of the potential fatal side effects of the trial and error. You must start with very low doses and work up to therapeutic dose/effect.

- ## 1. Tobacco

The active ingredient of tobacco is nicotine. Nicotine has a number of important pharmacological effects.

Firstly it is a muscle relaxant. This is from its direct effect on nicotinic receptors in the peripheral nervous system. It binds to the nicotinic receptors at the junction between the nerve and muscle and causes muscle relaxation. This is particularly useful in assisting the reduction of fractures and dislocations. If treatment has been delayed muscle spasms associated with the injury may interfere with reduction.

The spasm will both directly oppose efforts to adjust the position of the bone and contribute to the pain felt by the patient. In general, the administration of an analgesic and a muscle relaxant are indicated. Allowing a smoker to have a cigarette may help. In severe cases the use of a general anaesthetic is usually required. In the absence of other alternatives the following procedure may induce sufficient relaxation of the muscles to allow a successful reduction:

"A cigar is inserted into the rectum via the anus leaving at least a third of its length outside. If a cigar is not available, the tobacco is removed from 5-10 cigarettes and placed into a cloth bag, which is then inserted into the rectum so

that an end which can be easily grasped remains outside. Sterile water is used as a lubricant, and, if a bag is used, the contents should also be thoroughly moistened prior to being inserted. After 5-15 minutes, the muscles should relax sufficiently to allow a successful reduction. The insert should, in any event, be removed after no more than 30 minutes. Note that nicotine is toxic. At the first indication that the patient is experiencing any difficulty, the insert should be removed by gently pulling on the exposed portion. Safety in using this technique relies on the relatively slow rate of transfer of nicotine from the tobacco

leaves to the patient coupled with the ability to immediately halt absorption by removing the insert. It is therefore strongly suggested that no attempt be made to use an infusion prepared by "dissolving out" nicotine from tobacco. "

S Roberts. Personal Communication

Contents

Secondly it can be used to control some intestinal parasites and worms. For an adult, tobacco equivalent to that in 1-1.5 regular cigarettes is ingested. This should result in passing at least some of the parasites within 24 hours. For particularly severe infestations the dose may be repeated no sooner than 2 days after the original treatment provided a bowel movement has occurred in this period.

Nicotine is toxic and some individuals are particularly susceptible to its effects; if the patient shows indications of susceptibility to nicotine poisoning, a second dose should not be administered. Its effectiveness in clearing parasites arises from the differences in sensitivity to nicotine between man and many common parasites.

The primary problem with nicotine is the effect that produces the muscle relaxation also causes toxic effects, by activation of the nicotinic receptors in the nervous system.

A dose of 60 mg of nicotine will cause death in 50% of people who ingest it. The average cigarette contains 10mg of nicotine. While the amount of nicotine in cigarettes and cigars is relatively constant there is large variation in concentration in both wild and cultivated tobacco. As a consequence there is a serious risk of overdose. Like with Foxglove dosing is trial and error and using cultivated tobacco as a source of nicotine is potentially very risky and should avoided except in a major catastrophe.

Nicotine is also an effective insecticide and can be used as a spray on vegetables to prevent insect infestations.

• 1. Cannabis (Cannabis sativa)

This plant is deserving of special mention due to its widespread availability and use. Despite popular opinion it has very limited medicinal uses. Small amounts taken infrequently produce relaxation, a degree of sedation, and appetite stimulation. It also suppresses nausea effectively. Several studies have demonstrated that for patients with chronic pain, nausea from cancer treatment, or muscle spasm small amounts may improve daily functioning.

However, larger amounts and chronic use do have significant medical consequences, and for patients with pre-existing mental illness regular use can

worsen symptoms. Cannabis may be of value in the same way that any pharmacologically active substance can be, but this is not an endorsement of its recreational use.

• 1. Honey

While not technically a plant no discussion of botanical and herbal medicine would be complete without the mention of using honey as a healing agent. This is a common item in food storage programmes, but it needs to be in your medicinal storage preparations also. It is a very effective topical antimicrobial. It is easy to use but messy. It may also be beneficial in deep wounds and ulcers/bedsores.

Contents

Use: Pack the wound/ulcer with honey and cover with a sterile dressing. Change daily, cleansing the wound area with a strong solution of Echinacea root, repack with honey, then redress sterilely. Continue this treatment until the wound is healed. A real strong solution of Echinacea will have a numbing effect which will make the wound cleansing less painful.

This same treatment is excellent also for burns of varying severity. They will heal more quickly with improved skin regrowth. It may reduce scarring and infection.

Honey taken internally has also been found to be very effective in treating H. pylori which is the main culprit in the development of gastric ulcers. A tablespoon eaten every 1-2 hours for a week or so should clear up an acute condition, then a tablespoon 3 x daily for a week or so should clear up the condition entirely. A good maintenance dose would be a tablespoon daily.

- ## 1. Other medicinal plants

While there are many plants, which have medicinal, properties table 9.1 contains a list of some very common medications (not covered above) which are plant derived, and their uses.

Table 9.1. Other common medicines and there plant origins

Contents

Contents

| Daphne genkina | Yuanhuacine | Induces abortion |

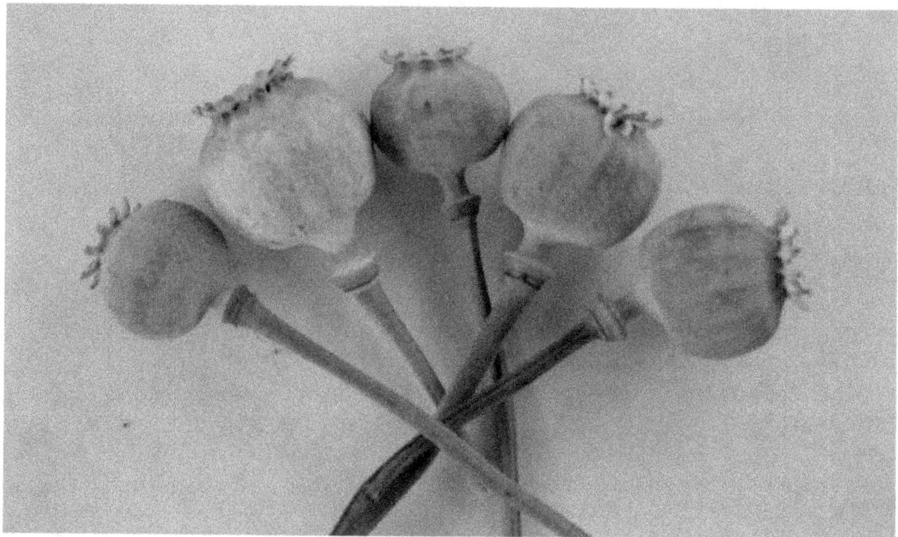

Figures 8.1 The Opium poppy. Morphine is derived from the poppy and is the mainstay of modern pain management. Poppy extracts provide the most practical option for managing severe pain in an austere situation. Beware: possession with the intention to use as a drug is illegal in many countries.

Chapter 9 Alternative therapies:

There is a huge spectrum of alternative therapies and associated practitioners. For the majority there is very little evidence aside from anecdote to their efficacy. A common underlying principle of most alternative therapies is good nutrition and a healthy lifestyle – the value of this is clearly not in dispute. How much of the remainder you choose to accept is a personal decision. A number of alternative therapies are based on scientific theories from hundreds of years ago which have been superseded by modern science. To accept these underlying principles requires you to suspend your belief in some of the fundamental concepts of modern science and especially physics.

Contents

It is vital you should take the time to look at the evidence for an alternative therapy or diagnostic modality before counting on them as a main part of your medical preparations. The weakest sort of evidence is anecdote and testimonials, and you should be very careful accepting any therapy that only has this level of evidence to support it. Also be aware of any therapy that claims it is too "special" or personalised to be submitted to the rigors of randomised controlled trials (RCT). The RCT is by no means a perfect way of assessing efficacy, but currently it is the best we have and the standard to which all medical therapies – conventional or alternative - should be held. However, a degree of common sense needs to be applied as well. Conventional medicine does not have trials proving every therapy works and neither should alternative therapies by expected to either. Some things we intuitively know are correct – you do not need a randomised controlled trial to prove that a parachute is better than nothing if you are about to jump out of a plane. The caveat to this statement is "that the rationale as to why a therapy works should make sense and not involve the suspension of the laws of physics in order to be able to accept it".

Colloidal Silver (CS)

CS is deserving of special mention because it is widely discussed in preparedness circles and many have a reliance on it for its antibiotic properties in their preparations. There are many anecdotes about how effective CS is in treating a huge range of bacterial, viral, and fungal infections, and many people have personal experience of its effectiveness.

Colloidal silver is silver atoms in solution, grouped together in clusters – essentially metallic silver in suspension – in an uncharged, non-ionic form.

Ionic silver has extensive antibacterial properties in the laboratory setting. There is a large body of evidence showing silver compounds (which release ionic silver) are effective topical antibiotics particularly in burns, chronic skin infections, and ulcers. There is no evidence that silver compounds are effective with systemic infections.

CS is metallic not ionic silver. There is no evidence that colloidal silver is an effective antibiotic. A number of websites make claims about the effectiveness of CS as an antibiotic, and one at least grossly misrepresents research which has been done.

The following articles should be read by anyone with a serious interest in CS:

1. D. L. Bowen & M. C. Fung, "Silver products for medical indications: risk-benefit assessment." J. Clin. Toxicol. 1996; 34(1):119-126.
2. Moyer, et al; "Treatment of Large Human Burns with 0.5% Silver Nitrate Solution." Arch. Surg. 1965 Jun; 90 pp 812.
3. Lansdown AB. "Silver: Its antibacterial properties and mechanism of action." J Wound Care. 2002 Apr; 11(4):125-30

CS is associated, if used frequently and in large amounts although exactly how much is an individual thing, with the development of Argyria (disposition of silver in the tissues) which is a grey or blue discolouration of the skin, mucus membranes, and/or finger nails. This is not considered to be a serious condition, but the changes are irreversible. There is wide spread belief that this does not occur with CS, but only with silver compounds. However, there are now a number of case reports – mostly in the Dermatology literature of this condition in patients using commercial or homemade CS.

Contents

In summary, there is no evidence that colloidal silver works as a broad-spectrum topical or systemic antimicrobial, and given what we know about how silver produces its antimicrobial effect we have no reason to think that at a molecular level it would work. This does not mean that it doesn't, but the absence of good evidence makes it less likely. The only way to know with any certainty is a RCT, however, it is unlikely that there will ever be any large-scale trials as such trials are expensive, and there would be no profit in one.

It is very popular and a lot of people have placed a great deal of faith in it. It is a risk/benefit situation – if you choose to rely on CS then you need to be aware of the lack of evidence and the real possibility that it does not work over and above the placebo effect.

The Placebo Effect:

The "placebo effect" refers to the fact that for any therapy a percentage of people will respond (it ranges from 0-30% depending on the therapy), and show a benefit that is not related to any pharmacological effect of the drug, and this benefit persists when a sham therapy is substituted for the real one. This effect is important in both conventional and alternative medicine. Despite the negative connotations associated with it, the placebo effect is a VERY GOOD thing.

It is important to be aware of this in an austere situation – not so much for you but for your patients. If you present yourself to the patient with confidence, and prescribe a therapy with confidence and conviction a significant number of patients will show

improvement even if you are only giving them a sham therapy – such as an alcohol based tonic – the value of this in a survival situation shouldn't be underestimated. The body is vastly more complicated than what we currently understand and despite its negative press if the placebo effect of a specific therapy helps people get better and is otherwise harmless (that's a very important proviso) then it is potentially useful.

Chapter 10 Medical Aspects of Shelter Living

While not everyone is planning on spending prolonged periods in a shelter for those that are there are 2 primary scenarios (with varying likelihoods depending on your point of view):

- Nuclear conflict – resulting in the need to shelter for a limited period of time (a few days to several months).
- Massive planetary change (climate change, comet strike) – resulting in the need to shelter for a more prolonged period (months to years)

Contents

The medical aspects of shelter living are an area that for many is neglected. One of the most useful points of references when considering the medical problems associated with shelter living is looking at the problems encountered on submarines or in the Antarctic. The similarities are obvious – enclosed space, cramped conditions, loss of privacy, potentially no natural light, same people day in and day out, and real or potential hazards. The people selected to work in these environments are carefully psychologically and physically screened so it is not possible to make truly direct comparisons with a shelter group, but we feel it is still very worthwhile examining the problems seen in those environments.

Psychiatric problems:

- 1. Boredom. This is likely to be a major problem even for only a couple of weeks and a major problem long term; combating boredom is going to be a major issue. A deck of playing cards and a couple of old novels won't be enough.

Research has shown that a human alone can only cope with 3 days of inactivity with limited stimulation before significant psychological distress occurs. This is seen in the form of loss of motivation, decline in intellectual activities (losing your edge), mood swings, and somatic complaints (headache, dizziness, nausea). The company of and interaction with others prolongs the period by several days. Several studies have shown that the average person needs 10-12 hours of activity per day to avoid boredom. Part of the answer is routine. Establishing a pattern, which occurs everyday, is really important for psychological well-being. People respond really well to having a routine and having clear jobs to perform. Everyone should be given an area of

responsibility and important activities that are theirs to perform.

Books, craft supplies, and games are vital to avoid boredom – catering for the range of ages which will be in the shelter. For children (and adults) structured teaching serves two purposes; reducing boredom and providing the opportunity for education about survival topics and issues.

- 1. Depression/low mood. Low mood will be very common depending on the situation. Following any catastrophic disaster there will be an immense sense of loss; loss of family and friends, loss of possessions, loss of usual routine, and loss of lifestyle. This will be on top of a background of high levels of anxiety over immediate safety, and security, and the future.

For the majority this will hopefully be relatively transient and be observed as a period of low mood and emotional lability. But they still retain the ability to function and over time improve simply with strong group support and encouragement. This sort of experience will be very common and entirely natural.

Contents

Unfortunately some will develop major depression. There is a formal diagnostic criterion for this but simply put it means someone with severe low mood to the point they are no longer able to function in their work or personal relationships. It is characterised by a pervasive sense of hopelessness, inability to concentrate, poor or excessive sleep, poor or excessive eating, and a loss of ability to enjoy things in life. Its management in a survival situation may be difficult. Its usual management is social support combined with supportive psychotherapy and/or the use of antidepressant medications. The majority recover over 3-6 months - some sooner and some considerably longer.

In an austere situation the most useful therapy will be strong social support. It is worth considering storing a supply of anti-depressants – especially one of the newer types such as selective serotonin re-uptake inhibitor (SSRI), the most widely known being uoxetine (Prozac) or a herbal alternative such as St. John's Wort. If someone is completely incapacitated or suicidal with major depression this may force some hard decisions on your group.

The above comments apply to any major disaster situation and are equally applicable to survivors not in a shelter environment.

- 1. Anxiety/Panic. It is reasonable to assume that some people may be so traumatised by their experience that they are unable to function or worse still they may be causing serious disruption to the other occupants. In stressful situations it is perfectly normal to feel panicky, anxious, or worried about things. The greater the magnitude of the disruption the more intense the feelings. It only becomes a problem when it interferes with there ability to function. For most people simple one-on-one counselling, reassurance, and the passage of time will be sufficient but for others it may not. You should consider your response if this situation did occur. Options include physical restraint, chemical relaxation or restraint (using psychotropic medication such as Haloperidol or Midazolam), or in a worse case scenario where the patient is unmanageable – expulsion.
- 2. Sexual issues. The issue of sexual tension also needs to be considered. The significance of this problem will vary depending on the structure of your group and the time you need to spend in a shelter environment. While you may dismiss this as not a problem for your group (and for a small family group it

Contents

probably isn't), please consider the following. If you confine male and females over puberty together (particularly younger adults) and subject them to large amounts of physical and psychological stress then sexual tension will develop, and sexual activity may occur; not necessarily between previously identified couples. This is a recurring theme throughout history; there is a high likelihood this will happen. For many, for religious and moral reasons this is unpalatable, and this has been demonstrated time and time again, and you need to give some thought to how you will manage it. Your solution may vary from segregation of the sexes to condoning the activity but don't pretend that this won't happen. Whatever you do it must be consistent in managing the overall mental health and moral of the shelter

- 1. **Privacy.** Privacy is also very important and becomes more important the longer you are confined. Allowing for an area in the shelter, if possible, which is partitioned off from the main living area where people can go to be completely alone and know they won't be disturbed will have a positive impact on mental health. Having the ability to have some "timeout" and privacy from cramped living conditions and other people will significantly reduce personal stress levels.

"Noise" privacy is also an important concept. Constant background noise particularly in a stressful situation can be a cause of friction and anxiety. This will be a major problem with young children particularly crying babies.

Controlling their boredom can control older children's noise. However, having a small baby crying for hours each day in a confined area will be extremely stressful. Consider options of a "quite room/space" with extra insulation, or earplugs, or muffs.

- 1. **Compatibility problems.** While not strictly a psychological problem, incompatibility problems between people in a shelter may become a major problem. Small groups form because of common goals and commitment. But a good relationship pre-disaster does not guarantee a good relationship post- disaster. There is no way to completely avoid this potential problem.

Have practice runs – can you still talk to this person after being locked in a shelter with them for 72 hours? Unfortunately often the first 10-14 days are relatively smooth – it is after that time that problems can arise. For those with a relative autocratic management style please be aware that while someone in authority is important for making the difficult decisions and having ultimate control, studies have repeatedly shown that peoples' psychological well-being (or moral if you prefer) improves rapidly when they are given an element of control over their lives. Giving individuals absolute control over what they do is not really practical in a small group survival situation, but allowing some degree of control for individuals will improve your group functioning and well-being.

Since most shelters will probably be based around family groups or close friends many of these issues may not arise and there will be a lot of support but it is important

to have thought about them, if there are any preparations you need to make, and what you would do to manage them if they arose

Infectious disease:

In a confined environment an outbreak of an infectious disease could be a disaster. Once you are established in a shelter the introduction of new bacteria or viruses is unlikely. Despite this outbreaks of infectious disease in submarines still occur after the incubation period for infections have passed. It is likely to occur due to 2 processes. Firstly from mutation of bacteria already in the body to a slightly different form, that is different enough to cause new infections. Secondly by contamination of the environment with bacteria and virus which normally live in the gut. Prevention of the first is very difficult in a confined environment. Prevention of the second can be achieved with fastidious attention to hygiene particularly with hand washing and food preparation. Disinfectant hand-gels are very useful in situations where water may be rationed. If you are likely to be in a shelter for the short-term, you should give consideration to using completely disposable plates and cutlery. One of the biggest sources of gut infections in primitive situations is the inability to adequately clean plates and cooking utensils. If you are planning for long-term shelter living you must ensure that the ability to hot wash your dishes with detergent is a priority.

There is no clear evidence daily wiping down of all surfaces with a dilute disinfectant reduces infection. Despite this it is a common submarine practice (those who remain undersea for months at a time) in some countries navies and they strong believe it reduces infections.

Light:

Light is important for several reasons. Day-Night cycling is important in maintaining a circadian rhythm. Loss of a predictable light/dark patterns leads to sleep disturbance causing somatic symptoms (headaches, aches and pains), increased stress, reduced ability to concentrate, mood swings, and erratic behaviour. Shelter lighting should be set to follow a day-night cycle with a predictable length. Over prolonged periods the pattern should be adjusted to shortening and lengthening of the light time to simulate changing seasons. This pattern appears to be relatively hardwired into our behaviour.

Light is also required for the activation of vitamin D which is required for proper bone growth. In the absence of exposure to sunlight or due to dietary deficiency adults develop osteomalacia (thin bones prone to fractures) and children develop Rickets which is characterised by weakness, bowing of the legs, and deformities of other bones. White light is not sufficient for this process to occur, and full spectrum (primarily UV) light is required. From a dietary point of view vitamin D is found primarily in fish oils and egg yolk. Supplementation with multivitamins is probably the best option for long-term shelter dwellers.

Exercise:

Contents

Exercise is important for both physical and psychological health. In the face of confinement and limited activity physical condition rapidly decays.

Space is likely to be at a premium in most shelter environments. If it is at all possible give some consideration to the value of storing small items of exercise equipment such as a mini-tramp or some sort of stepping device to provide the ability to undertake some form of aerobic or cardiovascular exercise. One possible option is using an exercise bike to run an alternator producing electricity to charge batteries or directly powering the shelter ventilation fans. Killing two birds with one stone, serving a very useful survival purpose while providing aerobic exercise. Depending on the physical shape of the shelter other options for aerobic exercise include skipping or sprint starts against resistance (such as a bungy). Anaerobic exercise is much for easier to perform with limited space using free weights, press-ups, and chin-ups, etc.

Exercise also provides an important activity of relieve from boredom. It should be built into the daily timetable as a scheduled activity and should be compulsory.

The importance of exercise has to be balanced against the energy expended undertaking it. This is particularly important in the face of limited food resources. If calorie restriction is in place then exercise should be limited

Nutrition

The excellent book "The Prudent Pantry" by Alan T Hagan is probably the bible for food storage programmes and we strongly recommend it or the associated Food Storage FAQ when looking at nutrition for preparedness planning:

http://athagan.members.atlantic.net/PFSFAQ/PFSFAQ-1.html

The key point relating to nutrition in a shelter environment is that relying entirely on stored food will be significantly deficient in several areas and if un-supplemented will prove fatal.

If you are relying on a very simple food storage programme with only the core staples then you will have problems quickly. If you have stored a broad range of items, and tinned, and bottled foods in addition to dry staples then it will be less of a problem. If you are in the former group as an absolute minimum you should ensure that you have an adequate supply of multivitamin supplements

If you are planning long-term shelter living you should give serious thought to developing a system for gardening within your shelter. Hydroponics is the obvious solution and can be relatively easily grown in a shelter type environment, however, it still requires large amounts of light, water, and nutrients to grow.

A simple but limited solution to the problem is sprouting seeds. This is straightforward – it requires warmth and a full spectrum light source. The nutrient value depends on the type of bean used, how long it is allowed to grow, and the amount of light it is exposed to. The more light and the longer the growth period the more vitamin A and C will be present with peak levels present at 8 days.

Unfortunately the peak palatability for these sprouts is 3-5 days.

In uncooked legumes (beans, peas, lentils) an enzyme which blocks the absorption of protein, is present. This enzyme is broken down with brief cooking. (Ref. The Prudent Pantry, A T Hagan, 1999 – no out of print)

Chapter 11 Long-term austere medicine

Introduction

Most of what is discussed in this book is related to a short to medium term disasters with serious disruption of medical services, but with a view to eventual recovery to a high technological level in the short to median term, certainly within a generation.

The above paints a possible scenario for what may happen in a major long term disaster – a complete permanent collapse of society and, with that medical services; no hospitals, no new supplies or medications, no medical schools, and no prospect of a significant degree of technological recovery. While this scenario is unlikely it is possible. Depending on your level of preparedness (or paranoia) possible scenarios include comet strike, massive climate change, global pandemic, or worldwide nuclear war any of which would result in complete disruption of infrastructure, and knowledge, and an inability to recover to today's modern level.

While all the principles discussed in other sections apply to the early stages of these sorts of disasters what happens when things run out for good, or the doctor/medic in your group is getting old, or dies raises a whole series of other issues. In this section we cover some of the main issues about long-term medical care in a primitive / austere environment. It is not a "how-to" chapter but more a discussion of likely scenarios and thoughts about what is possible and what is not.

Despite the pessimistic picture painted in the scenario above with planning and thought it is possible to maintain a surprisingly high level of medical care. We are not talking heart transplants and high-level intensive care, but we are talking quality medical care which can manage even if it cannot cure common medical problems.

Education/Knowledge

Knowledge is worth more than almost anything else. While at first thought it may appear that the loss of modern technology and medication will place medical care back to the dark ages it is important not to forget that the knowledge underpinning modern medicine is still there. While there may be no antibiotics for your dirty wound you still have an understanding of what causes infection, basic hygiene measures, and good basic wound care so while you may not have antibiotics to prevent or treat infection you will still know how to minimise the chance of infection, and optimise healing, and hopefully a knowledge of other substances with antibacterial properties.

Contents

In a long-term disaster it is vital that this knowledge is preserved. For this reason it is extremely important that you have a comprehensive medical library to begin with and that there is a priority to preserve the knowledge the books contain. It is also very important that the knowledge is passed on. There is always the risk that you as the medic may die. Having several people with detailed medical knowledge initially is ideal but this for many may not be possible. It is important that there is a degree of cross training within the group at least at a basic level. When it is apparent that a

disaster is likely to be prolonged it is vital that you begin to train someone to the same level as yourself; the best way is probably using an apprenticeship model over several years. This was the way the majority of western doctors (Middle Eastern cultures have had medical schools for the last 1500 years) were taught until the 17th century when the medical schools took over, and apprenticeships were still common up until early last century although they were considered inferior. Unfortunately learning medicine simply from a book is inadequate and having supervised experience in addition to books is the only real way to learn. For this reason if you are considering a long-term collapse ensure that you also have the resources to teach the basics of biological sciences first before moving onto medicine proper. It would be difficult to teach someone the complexities of medicine without a good understanding of the basics.

In addition to modern medical knowledge, if you are planning for a multi-generational catastrophe then you need to study medical history. The practice of medicine in the 18th and 19th Century provides, in our opinion, what we may realistically expect in terms of a technological level in medicine with our modern knowledge superimposed over the top. Look at how things were done, and with what instruments, what medications where used, and how; what were the medical problems encountered?

Much from that time is simply wrong and reflects the ignorance of physiology and pathology of the times but there is much to learn, and when approached with modern knowledge it is easy to identify what is useful information and what is not.

An interesting way to appreciate the medical problems of the time is by looking at the causes of death during that period; this gives some insight into likely serious medical problems in this sort of scenario now. Below are some of the commonest causes of death in early 19th Century in Australia. In addition to showing causes of death they also show some of the limited medical understanding of the time:

Contents

- Trauma (including drowning and burns) – deaths from drowning and burns appear to have occurred with frightening frequency. There were also a large number of trauma deaths – both as a consequence of (mostly) farming accidents and violence.
- Brain fever – while more recently (last 100 years) brain fever was a reference to specifically meningitis prior to this it referred to any high fever with a altered conscious state or delirium, so essentially any serious infection.
- Dropsy – the term dropsy refers to conditions resulting in fluid on the chest. While covering a number of different diagnosis for the most part it referred to heart failure and commonly followed episodes of severe chest pain although at the time this wasn't recognised for what it was – a myocardial infarction
- Abdominal distemper – this was a syndrome characterised by severe abdominal pain, abdominal rigidity, fevers, and death. A significant number of cases were probably appendicitis although it is likely that pancreatitis, liver disease (from alcohol abuse), and gallbladder infections accounted for a number of cases.
- Enteric fever – this was a very common cause of death especially among children. Again, more recently the term referred to typhoid fever, prior to this it referred to any dysentery.
- "Bubo" – This wasn't a particular disease but referred to skin lumps and hard masses in the abdomen which were associated with severe pain, weight loss, and death. This was probably a variety of cancers.

The ancient Egyptians also had a useful system of classifying disease and injury. They divided them into one of three groups:

- those conditions that can be treated
- those that can be contended with
- those that cannot be treated

It is simple but surprisingly useful because in an austere situation it gives a framework to classify what you can do for your patients; those you can treat and cure, those that you can palliate or make comfortable (until they die or get better), and those that you can do nothing for or where your intervention is likely to make things worse. You need to convey a realistic expectation to your patients of what you will be able to achieve and this provides a simple framework. There is no point is promising false hope. All you will achieve is your patients losing faith in you.

Lifestyle/Public health

Lifestyle: Prior to any disaster it is worth considering what you can do to improve your own and your group's health. Ensuring regular exercise, a good diet, maintaining a good weight, and that BP and cholesterol levels are monitored. Prevention of diseases such as heart disease, strokes, and diabetes is much better than attempting to treat them in an austere survival situation. You should ensure that all members of your group have their vaccinations up to date especially tetanus, measles, diphtheria, and polio.

Preventive medicine: A large proportion of the disease burden in the past is related to poor public health and preventive medicine. For the most part it was related to ignorance of the role of bacteria in causing disease. Key elements of preventive medicine and infection control include:

Contents

- Clean drinking water – uncontaminated by sewage and waste water
- Hand washing – soap production is a priority.
- Boil and filter water if purity not certain
- Sewage disposal – long drops or composting toilets and ensuring their drainage is not into the drinking water catchment
- Rubbish disposal – away from living areas, not draining into the drinking water catchment. Consider burying or burning what you can. Appropriate food waste into compost. You also need to consider how you will dispose of medical waste. Frequently this will be contaminated with blood and often infectious material. Incineration is probably the best option, followed by deep burial – away from water sources.
- Rodent and insect control – both are vectors for disease. Adequate rubbish disposal and trapping are probably the best methods for rodent control. Depending on climate mosquitoes may be a problem; stagnant water and rotting soft wood are foci for the mosquito larvae.
- Hygienic food preparation and storage – a large amount of food poisoning is a direct consequence of poor food handling and storage. Hand washing before any food handling.
- Isolation of anyone with a potentially infectious disease. Although many illnesses are infectious before symptoms become apparent it is important that any person who becomes unwell, particularly with fever or diarrhoea, is isolated immediately in an attempt to minimise further infections.

With diarrhoeal illness – simple hand washing is usually sufficient for the caregiver. With febrile illnesses or those with respiratory symptoms then barrier precautions should be used – gloves, gown, facemask (N95), and goggles should be used. If this level of protection is not possible then some form of face mask is needed when with the patient and hand-washing, changing clothes (hot wash), and showering before contact with the healthy.

Contents

For strangers arriving particularly during a pandemic consider 10-14 days isolation, followed by clothes burning and a through wash with soap before entering the community. There are no current infectious diseases with longer incubation times than 10-14 days. Provided the newcomer is symptom free at the end of this period you should be safe. This approach does not offer protection against those people who are carriers. However, among the current potential pandemic causes there are not currently carrier states although this needs to be considered.

The recent tsunami in southern Asia clearly demonstrates how quickly public health can break down. Despite widespread knowledge even in developing third world countries about the basic principles of public health and hygiene latrines have been dug next to water supplies, water wasn't being boiled, and in some places no effort was made to burn or dispose of rubbish, and it was just allowed to accumulate. While you can argue that some of this was due to "shell shock" from the disaster itself it just goes to show how the fundamentals can go out the window in a stressful situation.

Assessment

Assessment of a patient has 3 components – history taking, clinical examination, and investigations. At present there is a heavy reliance on investigations; in a long-term austere situation history and examination will come into their own again.

History taking and Examination:

With very limited access to investigations the importance of clinical examination will again take on enormous importance. While modern doctors are competent at physical examination there is heavy reliance on special tests, and many of the skills of accurate physical examination have faded. The basics are easily learned from any clinical skills textbook (We recommend Talley and O'Connor, Physical Examination) and with a little practice. With more exposure and experience you will be able to elicit more information. It is almost certain that in long-term austere situations that physical examination will come into its own again. The history 95% of the time is all that is required to know exactly what is going on. The examination and investigations may be used to confirm your thoughts, but it's the history that usually gives you the diagnosis.

Investigations:

Laboratory tests: Lab tests which are possible in an austere environment are discussed in the Laboratory chapter. These include basic urine analysis, blood typing, and cross matching, and simple cell counts. The minimum requirement is a microscope and slides. It is important to note that well cared for microscopes will last 100s of years.

X-rays: These will not be available in the austere situation. One of the main uses of simple x-rays is in the diagnosis of fractures. There are several low-tech ways that are reasonably accurate in diagnosing fractures.

Fractures of the long bones (tibia, fibula, femur, humerus, clavicle, ribs, etc), can be diagnosed by either percussion, or a tuning fork, and a stethoscope. Using a tuning fork is more accurate. A bony prominence on one end of the bone in question is tapped, or the base of a vibrating tunning fork is placed against it, and the stethoscope is applied to the other end. This is done bilaterally and the two sides compared. If a fracture exists on one side and not the other the gap in the bone at the fracture site will result in less sound being transmitted so the sound will be somewhat muted on the side of the fracture. Some specific points and caveats should be noted:

Sound waves will cross joints. For percussion finger or toenails can be tapped. To diagnose a hip fracture the sound source is applied to the patella (knee cap) and the stethoscope applied over the pubic symphysis.

The technique is less effective on the obese as fatty tissue will absorb sound waves.

Bi-lateral fractures can result in false negatives.

A 128 MHz tuning fork should be used as frequencies above this will tend to jump fracture gaps.

For long bones running near the surface of the body a fracture can be localized by drawing the tuning fork along the bone slowly (>30 sec, but <60 sec) until a very localized source of pain is identified (<3 cm).

Compacted bone ends of a fracture can result in false negatives.

A cone formed from rolled paper can act as a substitute for a stethoscope but is less than ideal.

Once again, the reality will be that the most useful method for diagnosing fractures will be clinical examination. This is also the case for the clinical chest examination in patients who would previously have had a chest x-ray.

Treatment

The trick to learn for patient care in a truly austere situation is to do what you can do extremely well. You may not have access to many medications or much equipment but do what you are able to do well and you will save lives. Basic hygiene and basic nursing care don't require much to be done well. The classic survival cliché is a simple scratch could result in you dying from gangrene infection of the leg. While at the extreme end of the spectrum this may be true cleaning the wound with copious amounts of water and keeping it covered will prevent most infections; if there are signs of infection further good basic wound care, resting the limb, and keeping it elevated for 48-72 hours will further the chances of serious infection all without antibiotics. Now obviously sometimes antibiotics will be lifesaving but you can reduce the reliance on high tech treatment by doing low tech treatments well.

Medical supplies/Instruments

Contents

Bandages and Dressings: Any absorbent material may be used as a dressing and any length of material for a bandage. It would be wise to identify what you plan to use in advance and ensure you store it. Wool when washed free of lanolin is very absorbent and is one possibility.

Table one contains an option for making and sterilising your own bandages. Here are several additional references:

- Special Forces Medical Handbook - ST 31-91B (commercially available), p578-80 discusses and illustrates how to convert finished cloth into dressings.
- Medical and Hygiene Textile Production; A Handbook - that is available from here: http://www.styluspub.com/Books/Book...productID=45873 .

This book takes a different perspective as it looks at production starting with raw materials and goes through fibre processing, spinning, weaving, bleaching, and finally

sterilizing, and converting into medical textiles. The level of technology is that of the developing world, and the illustrations could be used by the average person to build looms, etc. Coverage of turning finished cloth into medical textiles is not as complete, but offers a different perspective from the first reference. For long term autonomy from supply chains this is the book to have.

The primary problem with dressings will be with sterility. Provided the material used for dressings is clean, in most cases this will have very little impact on the incidence of infection. If you require a higher degree of sterility boiling your dressing material and then air-drying prior to use is an option – not perfect but this will give you a degree of sterility.

Haemostatic dressings: It is worth noting that TraumaDex is nothing more than purified potato starch and HemCon purified shrimp shell derivative ground up and placed in a bandage matrix. While we couldn't condone manufacturing your own it does give you something to think about.

Syringes and needles: Plastic syringes and needles are readily available and relatively cheap. If possible you should purchase as many of these as possible. While designed to be disposable plastic syringes can be reused; they should be thoroughly cleaned and resterilised by boiling. It may be possible to do this several times before the rubber and plastic degrades. Before sterilizing syringes that you are reusing, soak them in a solution of dishwashing detergent or soapy water

Needles, again, can potentially be reused but it can be difficult; all blood and tissue debris needs to be removed from the inside of the needle using a fine piece of wire from the top down, they may need to be straighten at the end, and the tip resharpened. They can be resterilised by autoclaving, boiling, or soaking in bleach.

More information on reusing and sterilising syringes and needles can be found in Chapter 6.

Contents

It is important to realise that the above advice is for extreme emergencies only. and it may be difficult to completely resterilise needles and syringes, and this leaves a risk of transmission of viral diseases.

The ability to manufacture syringes and needles is likely to be severely limited. It will certainly be possible to manufacture syringes if you have access to a glass blower – they are technically not difficult to make at least in a crude form. Needles, unfortunately, are potentially a different story. Even a good blacksmith will have great difficulty manufacturing fine needles. It may be possible to manufacture larger needles and cannula but they too are likely to be very crude. Alternatives to consider include bird quills and those made from blown glass.

The ideal situation is to try and obtain glass syringes and old-fashioned needles which can be reused and resharpened. They are surprisingly easily available from antique shops, auctions, and e-bay.

Table 1. Homemade dressing manufacture

Making your own sterile dressings:

Save Money by making your own dressings from old sheets or similar material. Here's what you will need:

- o White material for dressing (100% cotton is most absorbent)
  - o Colored material can be used for the bandage tails, if desired.
  - o Sewing machine
  - o Aluminium foil
  - o Oven

Cutting and Folding Dressings

Wash and dry material.

For a 2"x 2" dressing, cut a square of white fabric 6"x 6" square. For a 3"x 3" dressing, cut a square of white fabric 9"x 9" square. For a 4"x 4" dressing, cut a square of white fabric 12"x 12" square. For a 6"x 6" dressing, cut a square of white fabric 18"x 18" square.

For a 12"x 12" dressing, cut a square of white fabric 36"x 36" square.

These squares must be folded into thirds both ways to form a square dressing. Example:

6" Fold Lines 4" 2"

Contents

2" 2"

Fold

Fold

Fold

Fold

Fold

Fold

6" 2"

Step 1 Step 2 Step 3 Step 4 Step 5

For combination dressing and bandages:

Make the tails 36-48 inches long and the width equal to the size of the dressing you are making. Place the dressing in the middle of the tail and stitch on each edge or down the middle of the square dressing.

2",3",4",6",12"

Wide

Cut

Stitch

Tail (36"- 48")

For triangle bandages:

Dressing

Contents

Cut a triangle 55" across the base and from 36-40 inches along the sides. These bandages will last longer if they have narrow hem. (There is no need to sterilize this bandage.)

55"

Preparing for Sterilization

Bandages must be carefully wrapped in aluminum foil and protected from damage. They will remain sterile unless the foil is torn, punctured, or opened. The following are suggestions to minimize the amount of foil you might use:

For a 2" x 2" dressing, fold in half and place in a 4" x 4" piece of foil. For a 3" x 3" dressing, fold in half and place in a 6" x 8" piece of foil. For a 4" x 4" dressing, fold in thirds and place in a 6" x 7" piece of foil.

For a 6" x 6" dressing, fold in thirds one way and in half the other and place in an 8" x 8" piece of foil. For a 12" x 12" dressing, fold in thirds both ways and place in a 12" x 12" piece of foil.

The combos will require a larger piece of foil.

Sterilization

Place the wrapped dressings and combos in a pan or cookie sheet and bake at 350□ for 3 hours. When cooled, store in a plastic bag for protection, keeping sizes separate for convenience. Label each dressing and combo. They may be labelled with just one number, if desired. For example: For a 2" x 2" bandage, label it 2. For a 2" x 2" combo, label it 2C. Example:

Unacknowledged internet text file.

2 2C

Surgical Instruments: When buying surgical instruments it is tempting to purchase the cheapest you can find. This approach is fine if you are anticipating only using them half a dozen times. After that the scissors will lose their edge and be impossible to sharpen, the needle holders will begin to let the needles twist, and the forceps ratchets keep slipping. Unfortunately, as with most things you get what you pay for. If you are preparing for a long-term scenario then you need to invest in good quality equipment, otherwise, they won't last the distance. Good quality instruments will last longer than you will. The top quality equipment is designed to be reused in a hospital several thousand times and still work well – this is more often than you will use them in a hundred years!

Contents

The other option is the manufacturing of your own instruments. A good metal worker will be able to create instruments to a high standard but it very unlikely that they will ever match good quality pre-crash instruments. This also assumes that you will have access to a craftsman and a forge but it is potentially an option.

Many instruments can be improvised. Scalpel blades can be manufactured from thin pieces of steel – provided it they be sharpened to hold an edge. Dental extraction forceps can improvised from pliers. Many automotive tools are very similar to some medical instruments, and provided they are cleaned and sterilised may function well.

Suture material and needles: Most suture (particularly the non-absorbable) material will keep for a very long time. So, again, the ideal situation is to stock up in advance or scavenge. Alternatives to commercial sutures are discussed in the Wound Closure section. As with instruments it is likely a competent metal worker will be able to produce a reasonable range of suture needles.

"Gut" was the original surgical suture material. It is not exactly gut, it is the muscular layer stripped from the wall of the small bowel of sheep's intestines and preserved in alcohol. Cotton thread can be used both for skin suturing and internal sutures (even though it is not absorbable it can be left in place). It can be sterilized by wrapping it around a 1cm/0.5in rubber tubing and immersing in boiling water for 20 minutes, and used while it is still wet. Make sure the thread you use has a breaking strength of more than 1.5 kg/3 lbs by hanging an appropriate weight from a 10 cm/4 in long strand. If it doesn't bear the weight double or triple strands can be used. Avoid using this for interrupted sutures where possible.

Other equipment and supplies:

The trick with improvising medical equipment is ingenuity. Always look at what you have and think, "What else can I do with this?" For example, urethral catheters can be used as a catheter, or as a chest drain, or to control a severe bleeding nose, or as a cannula in an IV cutdown; a safety pin can pin bandages, open an airway by pinning the tongue to the lips, close a wound, remove a foreign body, or pop an abscess. Many items of medical equipment have multiple uses some are a poor second choice to proper equipment, others do a first class job; the key is think broadly about possible uses.

It is also important to realise that you have a huge scope for do-it-yourself equipment.

Below is a list of just a couple of ideas for improvised equipment but it's just a starting point, there is vast potential:

Splints – For a fracture to heal it needs to be immobile, and comfortable, and not cause pressure points. Plaster of Paris and fibreglass have been used for most long- term splinting for the last decades. Splints can be manufactured from just about anything that can immobilise a fracture site. Wood, plastic, strips of material, spun wool all in various combinations can be used to construct an adequate splint for a limb. One author has previously manufactured a perfectly workable traction splint for a broken femur from fencing wire, duck tape, and some insulation foam.

Contents

Fly Trap – Flies are a major vector for disease transmission particularly of diarrhoeal disease. The key factor in reducing the number of flies is adequate waste disposal. But trapping can also have a significant impact on numbers. Simple flytraps can be made with plastic soda bottles (of which there will be thousands around for years to come, regardless of what disasters may befall us – given their slow decomposition).

However, these traps can collect thousands of flies which decompose slowly so you need to consider how you will dispose of them. Emptying the traps is one of the worst jobs on the planet. Details on their construction can be found at http://www.talcuk.org/free/html/flytrap/flytrap.htm

Asthma spacer – Moderate to severe asthma attacks are frequently treated with oxygen driven nebulisers which aerosolise the asthma medication and improve delivery of it to the lungs. Over the last few years volumetric spacers have started to replace nebulisers. These are small plastic cylinders with a mouth piece which the patient breathes in and out through. The medicine is sprayed into the chamber of the cylinder and the patient breathes it in. The concept is that if medication is delivered into a confined space it doesn't disperse so quickly so by having the patient breath in and out through the spacer more of the medicine is delivered to the lung. A perfectible useable Spacer can be made from a 2L plastic soft drink bottle; the patient breaths in and out through the mouth of the bottle, vent holes are cut in the base, and a hole for the inhaler to spray through on the side.

Medications

Modern medications:

While these will eventually run out it is important to realise, as is discussed elsewhere, that the expiry dates on many medications have little relationship to how long they are safe and effective. The following information is for entertainment purposes only, and we do not recommend relying on this information except in a life- threatening emergency.

As has been outlined earlier medicines tend to loose their effectiveness in treating a condition rather than actually becoming dangerous. Expiry dates simply reflect the longest period of time the drug companies are prepared to admit they have studied stability for. Several companies (probably most – but they don't own up to having the data) have stability data extending 5 or 10 years beyond the expiry date on the packet. It has been cynically said that expiry dates are more about marketing, turnover, and profits than about patient safety.

Common medications that appear to have prolonged (up to 2-10 yrs), safe, and effective usage beyond their expiry date based on FDA and US military work include:

Contents

- Penicillin-based antibiotics
- Ciprofloxacin
- Phenytoin
- Atropine
- Pralidoxime (2PAM)
- Diazepam
- Cimetidine
- Opiates
- Thiopentone
- Paracetamol (Acetaminophen)
- Normal saline
- Lactated Ringer's

Synthesis of drugs

There are a several common and important medications that are relatively easily synthesised, and a number of others for which low tech synthesis is theoretically possible, but technically very challenging, and labour and time consuming. The requirements, aside from knowledge and time, are access to basic high school level laboratory equipment (there is also plenty of room to substitute things such as Pyrex kitchen bowls, measuring cups and kitchen scales), and some chemical reagents – which may need to be made themselves - the need to produce chemicals to produce other chemicals. It is likely that only a larger community could spare the resources to sustain a meaningful manufacturing system. We believe that community specialisation is likely to occur, and that medicine production (and medical supplies), and the provision of medical services may well be a desirable area of specialisation. The quality of the drugs produced will be significantly lower than current pharmaceutical standards; it becomes a risk/benefit situation in terms of using them.

However, safe, useable drugs can be manufactured Like other areas of preparedness this requires advanced thought and preparation about what you consider you may wish to manufacture.

* Simple Manufacture:

Alcohol:

Production of alcohol is very straightforward, we have been doing it for centuries. The problem is producing ethyl alcohol and not one of the many toxic alcohols particularly methyl alcohol which can easily occur. The basic process is well-covered in many books, and on the Internet, and is not difficult. It is useful for its antiseptic properties and also in the production of ether.

Contents

Ether:

One of the major advances in medicine in the 19th century was development of anaesthesia which gave the ability to perform painless surgery. Anaesthesia in the hands of an untrained person will have a very high death rate but in an austere situation potentially could be life saving. The first two anaesthetic agents were chloroform and ether and both are relatively easily produced. Ether is probably a safer agent and slightly easier to manufacture. Anaesthetic ether is diethyl ether – not to be confused with other varieties of ether.

The best way to produce ether is by dehydration of ethyl alcohol with sulphuric acid. When ethanol is mixed with sulphuric acid and heated in a glass distillation chamber (as found in any high school chemistry labs) it produces ether vapour which condenses to liquid. It has to be maintained within a certain temperature range for the reaction to occur. The process is essentially a continuous one with repeated addition of further alcohol. It is vital that the alcohol added to this reaction is ethyl (i.e. drinking) alcohol – other sorts will not produce diethyl ether and will be very dangerous. The sulphuric acid is reusable and catalyses the process.

Sulphuric acid is widely available, most commonly in lead acid batteries, and should be relatively easy to scavenge. During the Second World War Australian Prisoners of war in Indonesia produced ether with acid stolen from car batteries and home brewed alcohol. It can be manufactured by burning sulphur and saltpetre (potassium nitrite) together and while not complicated from a chemical point of view, it may be difficult practically although this process has been producing sulphuric acid for 400-500 years in very austere circumstances by modern standards. Of note is that mixing saltpetre, sulphur, and charcoal produces gunpowder.

The above description is only to provide the most basic of overviews and anyone considering producing ether should be consulting a reputable organic chemistry text. These substances are highly volatile, and the risk of explosion is very real. Also be aware that diethyl ether is a key ingredient of amphetamine production and as such may be illegal in some jurisdictions, and you may bring undesirable attention on yourself. It is also worth noting that chloroform is also relatively easy to syntheses.

Charcoal

Charcoal has a variety of medical uses the treatment of diarrhoea being the most common. The charcoal used in the treatment of poisoning (activated charcoal) is very different to standard charcoal, and while standard charcoal will absorb substances from the gut it is not very efficient. Charcoal is also extremely useful to burn in forges to generate the extra heat required to smelt metals, and in the production of black powder, and sulphuric acid discussed above. There are several methods for production which won't be discussed in detail here but essentially it is formed by the combustion of wood in a relatively oxygen-starved environment

Normal Saline

Contents

Normal saline is perhaps the most versatile of the intravenous fluids. It is extremely easy to manufacture. Standard normal saline consists of 1000 ml of distilled water with 9 grams of sodium chloride producing a 0.9% saline solution. The process needs to be sterile which may be difficult to achieve in a survival situation. The basic principle is the same as canning, and information on this is widely available.

In view of the borderline sterility of production, the finished product should be used within several days of production preferably within 24 hours.

Bleach

Bleach (a concentrated chlorine solution) is an excellent disinfectant of water, surfaces, and medical instruments. It is relatively easy to produce.

It requires a low voltage power source (12 V car battery is fine), a conductor made of carbon (or charcoal), a supply of water, and a small amount of table salt. The positive electrode is connected to the charcoal and the negative wire (with the plastic covering removed) is placed in the solution. The current is applied and chlorine is produced.

Details of the exact method can be found at http://www.pqs.org/ingl.htm

* Complex Manufacture

It is not possible to discuss the manufacture of these drugs in detail and below we just provide a superficial overview but it is included to provide some reassurance that limited complex drug production is possible.

Antibiotics:

Production of sulphur-based antibiotics, penicillin, and chloramphenicol in a primitive situation is potentially possible. However, the manufacturing processes are very labour intensive, require a long-term commitment from several people (potentially

taking labour away from more important survival tasks), some basic laboratory equipment, basic chemicals, and an understanding of simple laboratory procedures.

Sulfa antibiotics: These were the first antibiotics developed in the late 30s. They tend to slow bacterial growth rather than killing the bacteria outright so aren't as effective as those antibiotics that do kill bacteria. They can be life saving in severe infection slowing bacterial growth enough for the body's immune system to catch up. Their manufacture is relatively straightforward. The production of Sulphanilamide, the first sulfa antibiotic is a relatively common college-level organic chemistry experiment. It is well-described here:

Contents

Penicillin: In the case of penicillin the ideal situation would be to have a pure culture of the penicillase fungi prior to any emergency situation but this clearly has logistic implications. It is possible to isolate the penicillin producing fungi from mold growth but this adds another complicated step. The main problem is that a single culture will only produced 100,000-200,000 units of penicillin and this is about a third of a single dose. Multiple cultures will be required. Again, the key point is that low-tech production is possible but probably not viable for most communities.

Chloramphenicol: Chloramphenicol was originally grown from Streptomyces Venezuela. It, however, can also be synthesised from Acetophenone in a relatively complicated transformation reaction. However, with access to laboratory equipment and the right reagents its production is not difficult.

Insulin:

Unfortunately, there are a large number of people who suffer from diabetes and require insulin to control their blood sugar. There are two sorts of diabetics – Type I or insulin-dependent diabetics and Type II or non-insulin-dependent diabetics. Type I diabetics require insulin to survive. A small number of Type II diabetics also require insulin to have good control of their sugars but survival in the medium term may be possible without it using diet control and exercise.

Like the production of penicillin the production of insulin requires a lot of time, and labour, access to quality laboratory equipment, and an ongoing supply of pig or sheep pancreas perhaps several animals a week depending on the production yield. It is basic chemistry and like penicillin production is not challenging to anyone with knowledge of basic chemistry, but, again, the challenge is gaining access to the required equipment. What you produce will not be anything like pharmaceutical grade and will be much more immunogenic than current commercial insulin but it will potentially keep insulin-dependent diabetics alive in the medium term.

The basic procedure is fairly straightforward: extraction with 70% alcohol buffered to a pH of 1-2 with HCl to prevent digestion of the insulin by other enzymes from the pancreas followed by a five or six step fractional precipitation/crystallisation process

to get useable insulin. In reality any concentrated acid is potentially suitable. The process of crystallisation is aided by the presence of zinc.

Insulin can be extracted from many animals. Porcine (pig) insulin is probably the closest chemically to human insulin which is likely to be readily available. Sheep or cows are also a possibility, but the insulin is chemically more different to humans and, hence, more likely to cause allergic reactions.

A bovine pancreas yields about 75 mg/kg of insulin which assays at 26-28 IU/mg after purification, porcine pancreas a bit less, sheep yield only about 800 IU/kg but may be available in areas where other animals do not thrive.

Contents

We have deliberately avoided detailing the actual process as this information is freely available in medical and science libraries, but in view of the complex nature of its production the details are of minimal relevance to 99% of readers.

Thyroxine:

Synthetic Thyroxine is a medication required by some people with under-active or surgically removed thyroid glands. In contrast to insulin this can be administered off the hoof. Because there is less breakdown of thyroxine in the stomach oral administration is possible. Currently the need for and monitoring of patients on thyroxine is done using blood tests. In an austere situation the diagnosis would have to be made purely on clinical grounds which may be difficult. However, for those already diagnosed and on Thyroxine it is possible to treat them with sheep thyroid glands – several times per week – using resting basal body temperature as the baseline for treatment. Taking the temperature first thing in the morning before getting out of bed will show the subtle falls and rises in temperature associated with too much or to little thyroxine providing an indication of when to give and when to withhold the sheep gland. Again, this system is not perfect but it provides a possible solution for someone chronically taking Thyroxine.

As can be seen from the above examples relatively complex drug production is possible in austere conditions. However, nothing is ever easy – other chemicals are required for the process which may be just as difficult to obtain or manufacture, and certain items of laboratory equipment may be needed that are hard to improvise but it is possible. None of the above reactions are any more complicated or sophisticated than the manufacture of methamphetamine and amateur chemists in big cities and rural areas all over the world are cooking this! The above medications can be manufactured with 16th or 17th Century levels of technology with relative ease, and simply with 18th Century levels – it will all depend on how far back we descend.

Plants

In a sustained long-term disaster medications derived from plants and the limited range which can be easily synthesised will essentially be the only medications

available. Traditionally plants have been our main source of medicines and in the event of a long-term event they will be so once again.

It is important to be aware of which plant-based medications have clearly proven clinical efficacy and which only have anecdotal effectiveness. It is a current problem with botanical medicine that only a minority of therapies have proven benefit. That is not to say that many more are not very effective but only that there is no evidence for their use aside from anecdotes and case reports, but in a long term situation using plant-based medications with limited evidence (combined with a placebo effect) may be the only option. You will need to adopt the old traditional approach of trial and error in determining effectiveness and dose. Herbal and botanical medicine is addressed in much more detail in Chapter 8.

Surgery

Contents

Surgery has evolved to where it is today due to two fundamental discoveries – first the ability to give an anaesthetic and secondly the ability to sterilise and disinfect instruments and make the part of the body we are operating on as clean/sterile as possible. Obviously there have been thousands of other advances but these two alone are responsible for the other advances being able to occur.

With an understanding of antisepsis and the ability to give an anaesthetic (such as ether or chloroform – discussed above) then it is likely a reasonable number of basic surgical procedures could be possible. Such as limb surgery – amputations, washing out wounds and compound fractures, setting fractures; abdominal surgery – appendicectomy, caesarean section, very simple bowel repair in penetrating injuries and abdominal washouts; and a number of other "minor" major operations. It is also important to realise that lay people with a basic medical knowledge and access to a good book are more than capable of performing many surgical operations. If the alternative is death then making an informed honest attempt isn't wrong. This has to be tempered with the first rule of medicine: "First do no harm", whatever you do you shouldn't make the situation worse.

In terms of wounds and contamination - "The key to pollution is dilution" – for any wound or incision copious irrigation with sterile normal saline or sterile water if saline is unavailable will greatly reduce the incidence of infection. It's easy to do and it works. This alone will drastically reduce the incidence of infections in any patient unfortunate enough to need surgery in this sort of situation. Irrigation under pressure (the ideal is about 10 psi) will remove significantly more dirt than plain irrigation.

Some things to consider for surgery include: Lighting for operations:

The body provides many deep dark cavities which without adequate lighting are difficult to visualise or work in. If you are doing anything more than repairing a very superficial wound (and even then it helps) you will need good lighting. You need to see exactly what you are doing and the recesses of the body are pretty dark.

If you have access to electric power then overhead lighting or directed light with torches (flashlights) is ideal. The ability to focus light into the wound using reflectors also improves visibility. Head mounted touches are ideal as you can direct the light where you are looking.

Natural light frequently is more of a hindrance than help. Direct sunlight dries out tissues and causes damage especially for delicate structures like the bowel. Daylight can be good but not direct sunlight.

Working with artificial light from candles or oil lamps isn't ideal. It can be optimised in several ways. Firstly by directing some of the light into the wound using mirrors (roof mounted or small ones mounted on the surgeon's forehead to direct the reflected light) or reflectors behind the light source. Secondly by darkening the whole operating theatre and focusing the light around the operating area you improve visibility significantly. Using glass jars and bottles filled with water in theory can focus/concentrate light – however there is so much variation – depending the type of glass and internal and external curvatures that this often isn't helpful.

Ether Anaesthesia:

Contents

***The following is given for interest only – if you attempt to administer an ether* anaesthetic without the appropriate training – YOU WILL KILL SOMEONE**

The classic route of administering ether is using the "open-drop" technique. It is administered by dripping the ether onto a gauze square or piece of absorbent material held over face by a wire frame to prevent direct contact of the ether with the skin and to facilitate airflow. Ether is a solvent and contact with the skin or eyes can cause serious burns. The patient's face and eyes should be covered with gauze to protect them – if available Vaseline should be applied to exposed skin.

One common ether mask was the Schimmelbusch mask (figure 1); this provides an example of what we are aiming for in making an improvised mask.

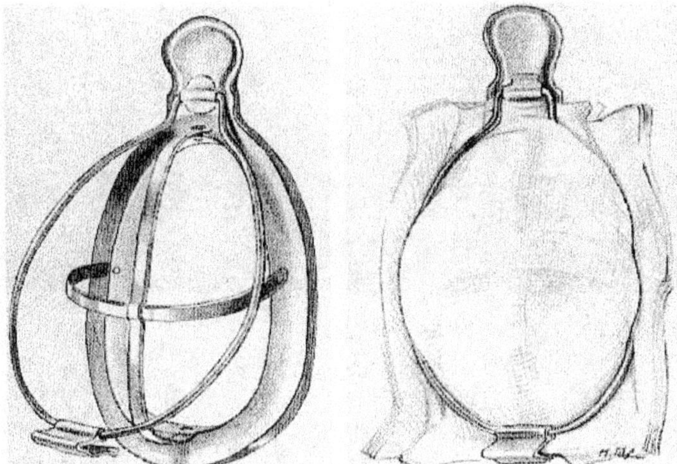

Figure 1. Schimmelbusch ether mask. (From a lecture hand-out of uncertain origin)

An improvised mask can be made with a small kitchen strainer (an ideal size will just fit over the mouth and nose) or you can manufacture a similar frame using medium gauge wire.

The ether is poured onto the gauze (you would need multiple layers) – the gauze should be saturated with ether. The gauze may need to be changed frequently as when the ether evaporates off as it causes "frost" to form on the gauze interfering with its effectiveness.

Contents

Gauging the depth of anaesthesia with ether is an art in itself – when is the patient deep enough to begin the operation, how much to give them to keep them asleep, how not to give too much and kill the patient. This is A VERY INDIVIDUAL THING. But rough guidance over drip rates are given below (to give an idea of the pattern of increasing volume during the anaesthetic) slowly increasing depth of anaesthesia to reach a level where surgery can be performed and then reducing slightly as the body becomes more saturated with it.

Ether (drops per minute)	Time (minutes)
12	1
24	2
48	3
96	4-15
50	15-30
20-30	after 30

It is difficult to induce anaesthesia in an adult using the "open-drop" technique due to problems reaching high enough concentrations around the mask. This can be overcome by using an ether chimney. This is essentially a metal column which sits over the mask, holding the vapour at a higher concentration close to the face which increases the concentrations being breathed in. It is also worth getting the patient used to the smell of ether first as it is highly potent and can cause coughing fits.

Contents

It can take a considerable period for a patient to wake up after an ether anaesthetic. It is reasonable to stop administering it slightly before the operation is finished. Ether also causes excess production of secretions in respiratory system and this potentially can cause problems with breathing – where possible Atropine should be administered to prevent this from occurring.

Chloroform is an alternative to ether – it is also relatively simple to produce. It tends to give a much smoother induction but also can cause more cardiovascular instability. Less is required than with ether; with chloroform the gauze is damp, with ether it's saturated.

One of the major problems of working with ether is that it is explosive. This limits your options with light sources somewhat in that open flames are a potential hazard. You should optimise your lighting as described above. It is possible to use ether safely

with open flames if you have no alternatives by keeping the ether and naked flame as separate as possible and ensuring adequate ventilation. Provided there is air circulating the ether is going to very rapidly be diluted with the surround air. A certain concentration of ether is required to induce anaesthesia (about 5%) which exceeds the flammable concentration (about 1.5%), but high concentrations should only exist around the head of the patient. A safe minimum distance to exposed flames would be 50 cm in a well-ventilated room but the process still carries a small risk. Static electricity from the operating team also provides a potential ignition source and should be considered.

All in all – if you possibly can avoid using ether with naked flames – the risks probably outweigh the benefits.

The best references to ether anaesthesia in an austere environment are either the 1981 version of the US Special Forces Medical Handbook, Anaesthesia Chapter, or Primary Anaesthesia by Maurice King which also has useful information on IV fluid production in austere environments.

Physical therapy/Physiotherapy/Occupational therapy.

These therapies support medical and nursing care and are very important. Physical therapy focuses on maintaining and rehabilitating musculoskeletal function – stretching, massage, and muscle-strengthening exercises.

Occupational therapy is focused on rehabilitating people to perform the activities required to look after themselves – eating, dressing, and personal hygiene.

It is beyond the scope of this book to discuss either in great detail – but if your goal is to rehabilitate a seriously injured or ill person back to full function within your community this aspect of care cannot be underestimated. Most communities will not be able to carry many people who cannot contribute meaningfully to the group. The goal of physical and occupation therapy is to maximise a patient's physical functioning, and get them to a point where they can look after themselves, and contribute. If you have a group member who has suffered a serious injury or illness early on you should focus on what they are likely to be able to do and tailor their rehabilitation to being able to perform that role.

You also need to decide as a group how many people you can support who cannot contribute to the group and who may require significant care and resources to survive with no return. You may face some difficult decisions. Fortunately with therapy most people are able to perform some meaningful work to "earn their keep".

The only book we have found specifically aimed at Physical and Occupational therapy in an austere environment is Disabled Village Children by David Werner author of Where There Is No Doctor which is available as a hardcopy or online. (http://healthwrights.org/books/disabledvch.htm). The book is primarily focused on the rehabilitation of patients with childhood disabilities and diseases but has much to

offer regarding the rehabilitation of anyone who has suffered serious illness or injury

and the focus is on practice in 3rd world environment which translates well to an austere or survival situation.

Other therapies

Discussed elsewhere in this book (Chapter 17) and of potential use in a long-term austere situation are rectal fluid administration, honey, and sugar as antimicrobials and maggot therapy for infected wounds.

Euthanasia

We know this an extremely uncomfortable topic for many and for others totally abhorrent from a religious perspective but it does merit discussion. Death can at times be protracted, and extremely painful, and distressing to the patient and others. Modern medicine has for years focused on easing the death process with pain management and other medication to control symptoms. In a protracted survival situation you will need to consider your approach to dealing with death and the process of dying. In certain cases, such as a slow death from cancer, without access to reliable painkilling medication then euthanasia may be an option for some. You need to think about it.

What would you do if faced with that situation?

Chapter 12 Woman's Health Issues

Despite the fact that women have been having children since the beginning of time, and the constant push that "natural childbirth" is safer, and is the preferred method of giving birth compared to modern obstetric practices having babies is a relatively high risk activity.

Contents

The current first world maternal death rate (and this is not just pregnancy and birth related problems, it includes accidents as well) is about 1:10,000. The current foetal death rate is 1:1000. In many third world countries maternal rates of 1:100 and foetal rates of 1:10 are still common. If you work in the third world today you will see daily maternal and foetal/newborn deaths. In part this is due to poor hygiene and maternal condition as much as the process of childbirth in these countries. But even excellent low tech midwifery care delivered with excellent hygiene practices to a healthy well nourished mother will still have a significantly increased incidence of maternal and newborn deaths. While it is often overused modern obstetric care saves lives and its absence will be missed.

The perception of low-risk childbirth has only come about through the development of expert midwifery and obstetric care in the last 50 years. For the majority of women childbirth will be very straight forward but don't underestimate the risk. In an austere situation there may be good reasons to avoid childbirth particularly for women who have already had a caesarean section or a complicated pregnancy before the collapse. In addition, a new baby is literally another mouth to feed, a breastfeeding mother has a higher nutrient requirement, and the child will grow, and need an increasing

proportion of the food resource.

Contraception

Contraception is important; preventing pregnancy may be desirable for many reasons as discussed above – maternal risk or lack of resources for the child. As part of your preparations you should consider options for birth control. Both condoms and the oral contraceptive pill (combined and proestrogen only) store relatively well in a cool dry environment – like other drugs their effectiveness will decline beyond their expiry dates but how much and over what time period isn't known. When used consistently natural family planning is also a reasonably reliable option (http://www.bygpub.com/natural/natural-family-planning.htm).

Abstinence is also an option which can also be considered. However, this hasn't proved overly successful in the past so there is no reason to think it would in a stressful future environment!

As is the case with food storage in that you should "store what you eat and eat what you store" the same is true for contraception. You should stick with the method you know – a time of crisis is no time to be trying out natural family planning for the first time, when you have used condoms for the last 10 years. However, you do need to be aware of the alternatives.

"Do it yourself condoms": Condoms can be made from sheep's intestines. While you are manufacturing your suture material you can also whip up a few condoms. The basic process is straightforward. They can be and have been manufactured from the caecum of a sheep. The process is fairly simple; the gut is soaked, turned inside out, macerated in an alkaline solution, scraped, exposed to sulphur vapour, washed, blown up, dried, cut to length, and given a ribbon tie for the base. It was necessary to soak them to render them supple enough to put on and they weren't disposable. The alternative method from early last century was to dip a wooden mould into melted rubber, let it dry and set, and then roll it off.

Childbirth

This is not the forum to discuss the mechanics of pregnancy, labour, or delivery. There are many excellent books (see references) on midwifery, which covers this in detail.

Your medical kit should have the basic components of an emergency delivery kit:

1. Your brain and your clean hands. These are the 2 most important things. You have to keep your wits about you and be ready to help if Mother Nature is having problems. The trick is in knowing just when to leave everything alone and when to help. Cleanliness is CRITICAL. Post delivery deaths from all causes dropped 95%+ when delivery attendants, midwives, and physicians started washing their hands with soap.
2. Something to suction the baby's nose and mouth out with. Like a bulb syringe, turkey baster, etc. You can also finger sweep the mouth or in a pinch put your mouth over the baby's mouth and nose and suck gently.
3. Clean cord, cloth strips, or cord clamps to tie off the cord, and a sterile (if possible

– otherwise immaculately clean) instrument/blade/scissors to cut the cord. This is important. Neonatal tetanus from cord cutting with dirty instruments accounts for ¾ of all tetanus deaths worldwide. It's OK to leave the cord attached to and with placenta at an even level with the baby for a while until you can get a clean instrument if needed.

1. Gloves: Sterile are better but at least use clean unused exam gloves. If no gloves are available then ensure your hands are scrupulously clean.
2. Clean towels and pads, and blankets to wrap baby in, etc.

Pre-packaged sterile delivery kits are available for about $10.00 USD with all of above in them.

Do you know why they always run around boiling water & ripping up sheets in old movies featuring a delivery? The hot water is, of course, wanted for washing hands and instruments, but also hot moist packs can be placed against mom's perineum to help relax the muscles and tissue, and allow them to stretch easier with less chance of

tearing. This is a technique which is completely lost in modern obstetrics that works well. Also ensure that you have a hand basin immediately available for frequent hand washing.

Most deliveries are very straightforward. This is why the human race has survived for so long. More than 90% of all healthy women will give birth with no problems at all. This still leaves a significant number of women who may run into trouble. Problems are more likely to arise with the first baby, with older mothers, mothers with previous delivery complications and/or multiple previous deliveries.

There are several areas where problems arise; the following is just an overview of the more common:

Contents

Obstructed labour/slow progress: Midwives are experts at encouraging slowly progressing labour without medical interventions. Currently if labour fails to progress it is augmented with oxytocin or a caesarean section. When there is no prospect of vaginal delivery due to obstructed labour or malpresentation then there are two options for delivery: Forceps/suction delivery or caesarean section. Both require significant skill and equipment. The reality for most is that in a primitive situation this will be beyond the midwife; if the baby is unable to be delivered the mother will die.

Breech presentations: This is where the baby is coming bottom first rather than normal headfirst. The head is the biggest bit of a baby. During normal birth the head moulds itself and slowly stretches the birth canal to a size it can pass through. When the bottom comes first this slow stretching does not occur. As a consequence there is a risk of the head becoming stuck or the baby being asphyxiated before the head can be delivered. There are a number of measures, which are well described in the references aimed at delivering breech babies.

If the baby dies during the birth process they can usually still be delivered without endangering the mother's health.

Infection: One of the biggest killers relating to childbirth prior to the last century was infection. It is not uncommon today particularly with more complicated deliveries but fortunately it is very responsive to antibiotics. You need to pay very close attention to antisepsis, ensure that if possible sterile gloves are worn, sterile instruments are used, and if gloves are not available that you wash your hands very thoroughly with soap and water.

Post-Partum Haemorrhage: This can occur early (within 24 hours) or late. Late haemorrhage is almost always due to infection. Early bleeding is caused by failure of the uterine muscles to contract and close off the connection site of the placenta; lacerations of the cervix especially the anterior lip, vagina, vulva; retained fragments or pieces of placenta; abnormal location of the placenta during the pregnancy (like all the way into the uterine muscle); rupture of the uterus; inversion/prolapse of the uterus; bleeding disorders & coagulopathies (blood clotting problems) either as a result on inheritance or pre-eclampsia/eclampsia. The most common cause is failure of the uterine muscles to clamp down (atony), lacerations especially the cervix, and retained placental fragments.

The textbook definition of haemorrhage is more than 500 ml of blood loss although it has been shown that the average blood loss after an uncomplicated vaginal delivery is often in the 500-600ml range. Also note that vaginal blood loss is consistently UNDERESTIMATED by 50-100% so that if you think you lost 500 ml it's probably more. Blood loss after delivery is normal in this amount, and assuming that mom was healthy and not severely anaemic before delivery is not a problem. Also it is normal for bleeding to continue in small amounts after the delivery, and bloody mucus (lochia) can continue for some time. But continued bright red bleeding like a heavy period or greater amounts, increasing size of the uterus (womb), etc. is not normal. Post partum haemorrhage accounts for 5% of maternal deaths.

Contents

Treat for shock just as you would any hemorrhagic condition: Lay flat, keep warm, IV fluids if available, monitor vitals, etc. Palpate the fundus (the top of the uterus); is the uterus firm and small (so well contracted and probably not the source of bleeding), soft and small (possibly not well contracted – maybe bleeding, or soft and big or getting bigger (not contacted and probably filled with blood)? Use gloves and examine outer vulva & rectum for tears, examine inside vagina for same, examine anterior cervical lip. Bleeding will either be coming from a visible source, or out of the cervix with no visible tears and, therefore, intrauterine – coming from within the uterus.

If the cause of bleeding is an obvious external or vaginal laceration manage appropriately with a repair. Consult the reference sections for more details on the basics of obstetric repairs.

Most heavy bleeding occurs simply because the uterus will not contract or a piece of placenta is left behind. Nipple stimulation either through breastfeeding or direct stimulation releases the hormone oxytocin which stimulates contractions and is the first treatment choice. Gentle rubbing of the fundus also stimulates contractions and should be tried. If large and soft, firm pressure on the fundus may expel accumulated blood clots and assist contraction. Also encourage or assist the mother to empty her bladder as this helps the lower part of the uterus to contract.

The second priority is to ensure the placenta is delivered if it hasn't been already and that it is complete. If the placenta is still inside or incomplete and bleeding continues to be heavy consider exploring inside uterus with a gloved hand for the retained placenta or pieces of placenta. You can also assess for inversion or uterine tear – this is very painful for mom if no anaesthesia is available, and there is a significant infection risk. Broad-spectrum antibiotics should be given if available.

If the uterus is empty and will not contract with nipple stimulation or rubbing of the fundus then bimanual compression should be considered. One hand is placed inside the vagina and the other hand is used to compress the uterus from the outside down onto the hand the vagina. This is painful and also carries an infection risk but can be life saving. Ice water lavage may also help slow bleeding – do this just like an enema.

If medications are available then oxytocin or ergotamine are powerful stimulators of uterine contraction and should be used if your nipple stimulation and fundal rubbing fail. Ergotamine is a derivative from the rye fungus ergot (Claviceps purpurea). Historically midwives used to give the black mouldy rye infected with this fungus to a woman who was labouring slowly or who had post-partum bleeding. The reality is that while ergot is excellent for controlling post partum haemorrhage if it is given to pregnant or labouring women it is likely to cause foetal distress and possibly foetal death. Like any botanical medication establishing the correct dose can be difficult and an overdose of ergot can cause vomiting, and severe hypertension, and possibly stroke.

Anything other than a simple repair job should be covered with antibiotics due to high infection risk.

Most bleeding will be controlled with patience, avoiding panic, repair as indicated, ensuring no retained placenta fragments, thorough uterine massage, and breastfeeding. It is terrifying to watch a post-partum haemorrhage; often appearing like someone has turned on a tap – DON'T PAINIC.

Contents

Whether this is an option for you is very much dependent on your skills and your ability to give an anaesthetic – either general or local. Untrained people attempting something like this even in an extreme emergency will probably do more harm than good and probably kill mother and baby. Obstetric anaesthesia is high risk even in the hands of an expert. A couple of general points:

- It is possible to perform a caesarean section under local anaesthesia (local infiltration as opposed to spinal or epidural anaesthesia) with and without sedation. How practical this is depends to a degree on the mental state of the woman. While removing most of the pain sensation, it does not remove the sensation of pushing and pulling associated with handling the internal organs. This can be a very unpleasant sensation for some women. However, evidence from Africa suggests that it is a viable option in a low-tech environment.

- The standard incision for a caesarean section is a horizontal lower abdominal incision then a horizontal incision over the lower segment of the uterus. This results in a stronger scar on the uterus and a better cosmetic skin incision. However, it is not the easiest approach. In an austere situation the skin incision of choice is a large up/down midline incision from just below the umbilicus to the pubic bone. Then an up/down incision over the body of the uterus, the so called "classical" incision. This approach is considerably easier for the novice from an operative point of view. Although the scar on the uterus is not nearly as

strong, and there is a significant risk of rupture if the woman subsequently goes through another labour.

Sympathectomy:

This is the surgical division of symphysis pubis; the joint connecting the pubic bones in the front of the pelvis. This enables the pelvis to open wider to allow the passage of the baby. The procedure is done from within the vagina under local anaesthesia. There is risk of serious damage to the urethra and bladder with this procedure if not done correctly and these are cut during the attempt. It can be life saving for the baby but has the potential to cause chronic joint pain in the mother and risk of infection.

What happens if the baby cannot be delivered?

Contents

If you have an obstructed labour or mal-positioned baby, and/or the baby is dead, and there are no facilities to perform a caesarean section then as unpalatable as it sounds, delivering the baby in pieces may be the only option to save the mother. If nothing is done the mother will die of sepsis. If the labour is prolonged with the head deeply embedded in the pelvis, pressure injuries can occur in the mother's pelvic oor, causing a fistula between the vagina and the bladder or bowel to occur – these are very common in third world countries and very disabling.

This is extremely unpleasant but can be done with a sterile wire saw and scissors. The baby's head is decompressed and then it is removed in pieces. This is rarely required and is a last ditched solution to save the mother, as in a major disaster situation with no conceivable access to health care. If not done in a sterile manner infection will be introduced and will likely prove fatal to the mother

"A Book for Midwives" by Susan Kline, Hesperian Foundation 1995 is the best single source of info on delivery, problems, and newborn care in an austere environment.

Abortion

This topic is offensive to many. If it is something you feel uncomfortable with then please skip to the next section. Unfortunately abortion has been a fact of life for centuries and merits discussion. Prior to legal abortion in the 1970s emergency departments on a daily basis saw young women with septic abortion and even tetanus from illegal abortion.

Historically a wide range of plants have been used to induce abortion on most continents and in most cultures. They have varying efficacy but most do work to a

degree. If this is interest to you most reputable herbal medicine texts cover this topic in varying detail.

Surgical abortion has been practiced for the last 200 years. It involves dilating the cervix and scrapping out the contents. Early in the pregnancy it is very straightforward. In the first trimester, psychological issues aside, surgical abortion is a very safe relatively minor procedure with a low complication rate. The risk of untrained people performing surgical abortions is high. Infection and perforation of the uterus are potentially life threatening and were very common in backstreet abortion. One point of view is that in an austere situation with limited access to medical care a first trimester termination, provided it is done in a sterile manner with appropriate instruments is safer than carrying the pregnancy to term. This is not the case, however, with second and third trimester terminations which if performed in an austere situation are likely to prove fatal to the mother.

Breastfeeding

An infant's ability to survive depends on its ability to get milk. For the first six months a baby only needs milk.

Breasting feeding is the Gold standard by a considerable distance for nutrition for children in the first 6 months of life. It is also the ideal survival food requiring no space or rotation and is readily portable.

Contents

The most reliable method of ensuring the baby is getting sufficient milk is their general contentment and steady weight gain. While there are many causes for irritable babies, when combined with poor weight gain it suggests inadequate nutrition. A common cause is insufficient breast milk although other nutritional problems can present in a similar fashion.

In the event that the mother's milk supply is insufficient or falling off there are several options. The first is the "wet nurse" concept. This was very common practice until the advent of commercial infant formula in the last century. If the mother had insufficient milk for the baby then another lactating woman fed the baby. There were women who did this as a career, and in upper class England this was common so the aristocratic woman could "preserve" her figure. In an austere situation this is only an option if there is another breast-feeding mother in your group either with enough spare milk or an older child who can be weened.

Secondly it may be possible to induce lactation in a non-breast feeding woman. Nipple stimulation to simulate sucking 3-4 times per day can lead to the onset of milk production after 7-10 days. This is more likely to be successful and to occur earlier in women who have previous had children and had breast-fed for longer periods.

In the absence of formula if a baby is unable to breastfeed they will die. If for some reason the baby is unable to latch on to the nipple it is possible to feed them expressed breast milk (EBM). This is usually done using a manual or electric pump, however, it is possible to milk the human breasts in a similar fashion to milking cows! EBM can

only be stored unrefrigerated for a couple of hours. It can be given to the baby via a bottle and teat or from a cup – even newborn babies are able to sip from a cup although this may take a little practice. They can also be finger feed – this is where you tape a very fine tube to your finger the other end of which is placed in the formula or EBM. The baby sucks on your finger and sucks milk up the tube – commonly used sizes are 6 or 8 French. Failing that a clean piece of absorbent material can be placed in the EBM or formula and then the baby can suck on this.

Commercial formula is an acceptable and safe alternative to breast-feeding. If you have infants or plan on having children it is important that you give some consideration to what you would do if you were unable to breast feed the infant. The unfortunate fact is that storing and rotating 6 months worth of infant formula may be prohibitively expensive for most and this is a risk you may need to live with.

In a truly austere situation it is possible to make infant formula from stored food although this is clearly sub-optimal. The following table contains several recipes for using stored food components to manufacture baby formula – please accept the caution that this is only for a life-threatening situation where there are no alternatives and the baby will otherwise die.

- 1. 1 x 13 oz can of evaporated whole milk 2 tablespoons of table sugar

19 oz of safe drinking water

1 ml liquid infant vitamins with iron OR ¼-1/2 adult daily multivitamin with iron crushed to a powder (a poor second)

Contents

Mix thoroughly, keep sealed, and use within 24 hours.

- 1. 3.2 oz dry whole milk powder 2 tablespoons of table sugar 32 oz safe drinking water Vitamins as in 1

Mix thoroughly, keep tightly sealed, and use within 24 hours

- 1. 3.2 oz dry non-fat milk powder 2 tablespoons of table sugar

3 tablespoons (28gms) of vegetable oil Vitamins as in 1

Mix thoroughly, keep tightly sealed, and use within 24 hours (The Prudent Pantry; Alan T Hagan, Borderline Press 1999)

Chapter 13 Medical Aspects of Nuclear Biological and Chemical warfare

While it is possible to survive an NBC attack any significant attack would result in serious medical consequences. The following chapter looks at medical issues relating to NBC attacks particularly focusing on small group issues. This is basic overview and further references should be consulted for more detailed information.

There are three subsections under each heading category: Prevention, Equipment, and Medical preparations.

Nuclear

Prevention:

Try to relocate to avoid living near a nuclear target such as a big city or military base. Avoidance of risk is the only valid prevention strategy.

Equipment:

The most important thing to have is shelter. We recommend "Nuclear War Survival Skills" by Cresson H. Kearny. (http://www.oism.org/nwss/).This book discusses several low-tech approaches to nuclear survival. Most of the equipment recommended is standard in most homes or readily available. The decision on the purchase of monitoring equipment is a personal one. If you have a formal shelter and long term supplies then there is probably a role for monitoring equipment. If you are using an expedient shelter it would seem to be logical that you stay in your shelter for as long as practical and if forced to leave only do so for brief periods. If you are forced to leave is there any value in knowing how much radiation you have received?

Contents

Medical Preparations:

An unsheltered person 1.5 km from a 1-megaton bomb could expect to receive about 500 rads of radiation from the initial explosion if they survive the blast and heat injuries. This level of exposure gives about a 50% survival rate. Simple sheltering from the initial blast significantly reduces this initial exposure.

Added to this is exposure from fallout (residual radiation) over the short to medium term. Issues such as the weather and ground or air explosion will have a big impact on dose of radiation delivered.

When considering clinical radiation effects they are broken down into:

- Immediate symptoms (0.5-6 hrs) – dose dependent
  Nausea, vomiting, loss of appetite, and loss of energy

- Symptom-free period (3 hrs – 3 weeks) – dose dependent
- Second phase symptoms (1-2 days to 3 weeks) – dose dependent. Recovery or death occurs in a further 3-4 weeks
  - GI symptoms – nausea, vomiting, diarrhoea
  - Bone marrow suppression – infection, bleeding
  - Cerebral and vascular – very high doses cause blood vessels to become leaky, and chemical mediators to activate causing edema (fluid leaking from blood vessels) and shock. The brain is very sensitive to high doses and this leads to confusion, seizures, and coma. Patients presenting with cerebral and vascular signs and symptoms will die over a 1 to 2-week time frame.

In an austere situation without access to dosimeters the timing of onset of initial symptoms, and the length of the symptom-free period enable you to estimate very roughly the likely exposure, and mortality, and provide a guide for triaging medical resources. Patients who present only with GI and marrow suppression symptoms, with a delayed onset of initial symptoms, and a long symptom-free period may benefit from intensive management with fluid resuscitation and intravenous antibiotics

Those with early onset initial symptoms and a minimal symptom-free period especially if they have brain symptoms and signs will die, and treatment is wasted on them in a survival situation

Cumulative exposure will give the following timing of initial symptoms:

<150 rads: Minimal initial symptoms only. Increased long term cancer risks. 150-450 rads: Initial symptoms can occur 1-4 hours post-exposure depending on

dose. Symptom-free period of 10-20 days. Deaths approach 50% at the top end of the range

450-800rads: Initial symptoms 30-60 minutes post exposure lasting 12-48 hours.

Symptom-free period of 2-10 days. Deaths approach 100% at the top end of the range.

>800 rads: Incapacitation soon after exposure, and death within 1-2 days with no symptom-free period.

Median lethal dose with no medical treatment is 350-400 rads.

Radiation is not the only effect of nuclear explosions. A significant number of deaths and injuries arise from other effects of the explosion.

Heat: The thermal wave generated from the blast can cause serious burns. If you are planning for a nuclear disaster then you will need to address the issue of burn management and stock your supplies accordingly

Blast: Injuries occur for 2 reasons. Firstly damage from the pressure wave itself – ear, lung, and gut injuries are most common, and secondly from collision with objects carried by the blast wave (wood, glass, nails), or the patient themselves colliding with solid objects when thrown by the wave.

Potassium Iodide: Radioactive isotopes of iodine can be taken up by the thyroid gland following a nuclear blast. This causes a significant risk of thyroid cancer. By

taking potassium iodide or potassium iodate supplement (approximately 76% iodine); the uptake by the thyroid gland can be blocked to a degree. The dose is 130 mg once a day starting before exposure and continuing for 10 days. Potassium iodate has been shown to be more palatable to children as it tastes much less bitter in comparison to iodide.

Prussian blue: The FDA has determined that the 500 mg Prussian blue capsules, when manufactured under the conditions of an approved New Drug Application (NDA), has been found a safe and effective for the treatment of known or suspected internal contamination with radioactive cesium, radioactive thallium, or non- radioactive thallium. This determination is based on a careful review of published literature articles containing reports, data, and experiences of people who were exposed to high levels of thallium or cesium-137, and who were treated effectively with Prussian blue.

http://www.fda.gov/cder/drug/infopage/prussian_blue/Q&A.htm#1

Other blocking options: While there is evidence to support potassium iodide and Prussian blue there is little evidence supporting other blocking agent. Russian scientists following Chernobyl have suggested that the ingestion of excessive calcium in combination with vitamin D may decrease absorption of radioactive strontium.

Strontium has a known affinity for bones. The excess calcium may be taken up in place of some of the otherwise bioavailable strontium leaving the rest to be cleared from the body without deposition. This is scientifically sound theory although there is no evidence demonstrating a benefit but no reason to think it would be harmful.

Biological

Prevention

Hygiene is the single most important step to prevention illness/death from the use of biological weapons or biological agents in general. This includes clean drinking water, proper waste disposal, and hygienic food preparation, cooking, food storing, and slaughter of animals. Make sure that you have strict guidelines relating to hygiene, and that everybody in your group understands and follows them. The other important step is to keep up to date on vaccinations.

Do a risk analysis of what you believe is the biggest biological threat for your group. Some infectious diseases (measles, polio, diphtheria) are returning because childhood vaccination rates are falling

Equipment

Firstly what is required for basic hygiene and cleanliness – brooms, dustpans, mops, bleach, disinfectants, etc. Secondly, specific items for dealing with infectious disease. Simple barrier precautions will protect you from the majority of infectious agents.

1. Hand washing
2. Mask: Varies from a simple paper mask to a full gas mask unit. Paper masks must be certified to the N95 or N100 standard. This refers to the filtration rate for a given particle size rather than the size of the particles themselves. i.e. an N95 is rated as filtering greater than 95% of all particles

1.0 microns or larger in size. These standards are effective for protection against many infective agents, not all (especially some viri), but they reduce the changes of inhalation significantly. If you purchase gas masks then you must ensure that the filter is against biological agents and not simply chemicals. The masks must be sized to the individual – find correct sizing needed before you need to depend on them.

Contents

1. Gloves: These reduce the degree of skin contamination but are not an alternative to frequent hand washing.
2. Gowns: These provide an additional layer of protection and reduce regular clothing contamination
3. Over-suits: A waterproof over-suit combined with mask and gloves offers the most complete protection. *Be aware though that the more complicated the personal protective equipment the more likely you are to contaminate yourself getting out of it.* Scrubbing down with disinfectant prior to removing your equipment, removing your mask last, and through hand washing reduce the risk further.

Medical Preparations:

It is not practical to keep on hand supplies to deal with all biological possibilities. So consider stocking up on what is likely to cover the most diseases. We recommend where it is possible storing ciprofloxacin and doxycycline. Also stock up on IV fluids and antipyretics, such as paracetamol (acetaminophen).

During a biological attack it may take several days to identify the agent but it is likely that early on you will know what you are dealing with.

Common Biological agents:

Inhalation anthrax

Symptoms: Short period with non-specific flu like symptoms. Often a symptom-free period then one–two days later patient develops high fever and shortness of breath often associated with coughing up blood

Primitive treatment: Doxycycline or Ciprofloxacin Inhalation anthrax is not contagious. High death rate

Tularaemia

Symptoms: Fever, shortness of breath, fatigue, malaise, cough, and abdominal pain. Primitive treatment: Doxycycline or ciprofloxacin

Simple barrier precautions should be sufficient as Tularaemia is usually not contagious.

Pneumonic Plague (Yersinia pestis)

Symptoms: Fatigue, fever, cough, shortness of breath, and malaise.

Primitive treatment: Doxycycline or ciprofloxacin

Contents

Pneumonic Plague is highly contagious, and caregivers need to protect themselves from droplets. Fleas on rodents also transmit plague zoonotically – keep the rat population under control and there will be fewer rats to spread the fleas.

Botulism

Symptoms: Blurry vision, difficulty speaking and swallowing, sore/dry throat, dizziness, and paralysis.

Primitive treatment: Supportive. Prolonged (weeks) mechanical/manual ventilation may be required.

It is not contagious.

Smallpox

Symptoms: Fever, rigors (uncontrolled shaking), malaise, headache, and vomiting. After a couple of days a pustular rash develops on the hands, face, and trunk.

Primitive treatment: Supportive

High contagious - both contact and airborne.

Viral Hemorrhagic Fever

Symptoms: GI bleedings, petechia, bleeding from mucous membranes. Primitive treatment: Supportive

Some VHFs are contagious. As a rule in primitive conditions assume all suspected cases are highly contagious.

Brucellosis (Brucella melitensis)

Symptoms: Fever, headache, sweating, chills, back pain Primitive treatment: Doxycycline + rifampicin

Usually nonfatal. Found in animal reservoirs in cows, pigs, goats, and sheep. Can be transmitted as an aerosol or through contact with body fluids. Second line biological agent due to low kill potential but has the potential to overwhelm medical services due to epidemic outbreaks.

Encephalomyelitis

Symptoms: Fever, headache, severe photophobia (aversion to light). Primitive treatment: Supportive.

Contents

Alphavirus infection (Eastern, Western, or Venezuelan Equine Encephalomyelitis). High mortality. If occurs outside endemic areas may indicate biological attack.

Meliodosis and Glanders (Burkholderia pseudomalleri)

Symptoms: Pneumonia with associated septicaemia. Meliodosis may occur in the form of localised lesions.

Primitive treatment: Ceftazidime for acute infection, doxycycline to prevent recurrence.

Normal infection occurs via contaminated soil or water in endemic areas. Dispersal can be via aerosol in a biological attack. This disease is endemic in northern Australia. Second line bio agent.

Psittacosis (Chlamydia psittaci)

Symptoms: Atypical pneumonia with fever and cough. Primitive treatment: Doxycycline.

Rarely fatal. Transmitted naturally to humans after contact with infected bird droppings. Second line bio agent.

Q-Fever (Coxiella burnetti)

Symptoms: High fevers, chills, sweats, headache. Primitive treatment: Doxycycline or Chloramphenicol

Human transmission usually from inhaled dust infected with placental tissue or secretions from infected sheep, cows, or goats. Rarely fatal. Second line bio agent.

Typhus fever (Rickettsia prowazekii)

Symptoms: Fever, headaches, chills, generalised pain and rash. Primitive treatment: Doxycycline or Chloramphenicol

Moderate fatality rate. Transmitted from infected person to infected person by human body lice. Second line bio agent

Ricin (technically a chemical agent)

Symptoms: Block protein synthesis within the body. Abdominal pain, diarrhoea, nausea, vomiting, severe diarrhoea. Pneumonia if infection by inhalation route. Cardiovascular collapse.

Primitive treatment: Supportive.

Contents

Derived from the castor bean. Highly potent. Inhalation following spraying is most likely route of spread.

Supportive Treatment.

The treatment of many biological agents is described as supportive care. This is the support of the body's organ systems (heart, brain, liver, kidneys) to help them continue to function following damage but is not specifically aimed at treating the underlying injury or disease. It is usually delivered in an intensive care unit and consists of treatments such as oxygen, ventilation, dialysis, fluid therapy, nutrition, and using medications to maintain blood pressure. This is in addition to antibiotics if they are appropriate. In an austere situation your ability to deliver supportive care will be minimal and potentially a massive drain on limited resources. Within an austere environment it may be possible to hand ventilate a patient for a limited period (prolonged Ambu-bag ventilating is extremely demanding on the hands, and in our experience a single person cannot do it for more than 20-30 minutes at a time), and administer IV fluids. But intensive supportive care beyond that is simply not practical.

Chemical Weapons

Prevention

The only prevention is avoiding exposure. Since it is likely any exposure would be the result of a terrorist attack it may be difficult to avoid. The best option is to ensure that you have access your mask at all times. Make sure you train with your mask and filter and can ensure it properly fitted. *If dealing with a patient of suspected chemical agent poisoning ensure you are protected and that the patient is decontaminated. Where*

formal decontamination is not possible – remove and dispose of their clothes and wash them down with soap and water.

If you suspect a chemical attack try and stay up wind from the location and on the high ground. Chemical agents will be carried by the wind and as most are heavier than air the chemicals will settle in low lying areas. Inside try and find a room with minimal windows (ideally an interior room with no windows), tape cracks around doors and windows and place a wet towel around the base of the door

Equipment

The single most important piece of equipment is a protective facemask and appropriate filters for all the members of your family. Ensure your filters meet the standard for both biologicals, and organic chemicals, and that you have spares.

Beware of military surplus masks; the quality in some cases is questionable.

The appropriate military filters will provide protection against chemical agents. Buying the correct civilian filter can be more difficult. The following is the Australian commercial standard for mask filters which is the most appropriate for this application: A2B2E2K2 Hg P3.

Contents

"A" protection against organic compounds with boiling point > or = to 65°C (Most nerve agents) "B" protection against Inorganic gases and vapors e.g. chlorine, hydrogen sulphide, hydrogen cyanide (most blood agents)

"E" protection against sulphur dioxide, hydrogen chloride and other acid gases. "K" protection against ammonia and organic ammonia derivatives

"2" is the filter class and means a maximum permissible concentration of toxic substance = 0,5%vol% (5000ppm)

"Hg" is protection against Mercury.

"P3" particulate filter at the highest class (most viruses + radioactive dust)

In the US, suitable commercial filters are "violet ring" (M95 particulate /organic solvent / radon) rated 40mm thread. The military spec is C2A1 Military Spec NBC filter with a NATO thread (40 mm).

The mask protects you from vapour and gas. A protective over-suit protects you from liquid and dense vapour contamination on your skin. Usually liquid does not spread over a wide area while vapour can disperse over wide distances. Vapour is poorly absorbed from the skin but it can be if the vapour is dense enough but this is only likely close to the release point. The need for skin protection is particularly a problem with blister agents. For most people the priority is the purchase of appropriate gasmasks before considering over-suits. If you are unable to afford commercial chemical protective suits consider purchasing those recommended for spraying agricultural chemicals; they do offer the same level of protection but are cheaper, and many nerve agents are based around organophosphate agricultural sprays.

Medical preparations

In an austere situation Tincture of green soap (or another mild soap) is still the recommended low-tech decontamination agent for suits and bodies. Obviously care must be taken decontaminating others.

Chemical weapons are divided in three types: Nerve Gas, Blood agents, and Blister agents.

Nerve gas: GA(tabun), GB(sarin), GD(soman), GF(cyclohexyl sarin) and VX Nerve gas can cause sweating, excess saliva, excess respiratory secretions, tachycardia (fast heart rate) or bradycardia (slow heart rate), abdominal cramps, vomiting, muscle twitching, headache, seizures, confusion, and coma. They cause

their effects by blocking the breakdown of acetylcholine – a communication chemical between nerves and muscles. When the enzyme, which breaks it down, is blocked, it accumulates, and causes the symptoms of nerve agent poisoning.

Treatment:

Contents

Pre-treatment: This consists of the administration of medication prior to exposure to a nerve agent to minimise the effect of the agent. This is only useful if the chance of exposure is high and there is some warning. The agent of choice is Pyridostigmine

30 mg every 8 hours. This binds reversibly to the same receptors to which the nerve agents bind irreversibly helping to reduce their effects. This was tolerated for prolonged periods by troops during Gulf War 1 with minimal minor side effects. If exposure occurs then pre-treatment combined with post-exposure treatment significantly reduces the death rate.

Post-exposure treatment: This should be administered immediately upon suspicion of exposure to nerve agents (i.e. high risk situation plus unexplained salivation, excess nasal secretions, shortness of breath, muscle twitching). There are 3 components:

1. Atropine: 2 mg by IM injection repeated up to 3 times in 30 minutes if symptoms are persisting or worsening. Large amounts of atropine may be required, but the indications and administration are beyond the scope of this book. The dose is titrated against signs of atropinization: dry mouth, dry skin, and tachycardia > 90 min. In the complete absence of medical care and confirmed nerve agent exposure atropine can be continued to maintain atropinization for 24 hours (usually 1-2 mg Atropine 1-4 hourly). Atropine effects are essentially peripheral and it has only a limited effect in the central nervous system
2. Oxime treatment: While atropine minimises the symptoms it does not reverse the enzyme inhibition caused by the nerve agent. By administering oximes this encourages the reactivation of the enzymes required to breakdown the acetylcholine. Different oximes work better with different nerve agents usually a mix of Pralidoxime and Obidoxime is given.
3. Anticonvulsants: In severe exposures there is the risk of seizures leading to serious brain injury. Atropine has a limited effect in the brain. Diazepam is the drug of choice and can be given 10 mg IM repeatedly to control the convulsion.

Patients with severe exposures may also require assisted ventilation and suctioning of their airways.

While pre-treatment and initial first aid treatments are relatively straight forward the ongoing medical management of patients exposed to nerve agents is complicated. If you do have access to the antidotes please follow a reputable NBC or toxicology references to confirm the advice above and find further information about ongoing management.

If you are able to get access to military autoinjectors then this is ideal first aid/initial therapy. There are 3 common brands of auto injectors:

Combopen (UK) 500 mg Pralidoxime, 2 mg Atropine, 10 mg Avizafone Combopen (Aust) 220 mg Obidoxime, 2 mg Atropine

Mark 1 (USA) 600 mg Pralidoxime, 2 mg Atropine

Pralidoximine is available in vials and in autoinjectors by itself also for organophosphate poisoning

Blood agents

Contents

The most common of these agents is cyanide or its derivatives. They work by blocking cellular respiration. It is mainly spread by aerosol. If the patient survives the initial contact then it is likely that the patient will survive. The spectrum of symptoms runs from weakness, dizziness, and nausea through seizures and respiratory arrest.

Treatment:

Remove from exposure area and decontaminate the patient.

There is no true austere management. Where possible provide 100% oxygen and assist with ventilation (this is the single most useful step). There are 3 options for therapy:

1. Hydroxycobalamine: 5 gms IV – safest therapy
2. Amyl nitrite (inhaled – usually a temporising measure until IV medication can be given) or sodium nitrite 300 mg IV over 10 minutes followed by sodium thiosulphate 12.5 gm over 15 minutes. This combination forms the commonly available "Eli Lily kit"
3. Dicobalt edetate 600 mg followed by sodium thiosulphate – very toxic therapy and least ideal of the three.

Blister agents

Blister agents include Lewisite and Mustard gas. These cause damage to the skin and when inhaled damage to the lungs. Mustard gas can also cause suppression of the bone marrow; if this occurs in an austere situation death is likely from infection.

Treatment:

Protecting yourself from contamination is the first priority. Decontaminate the patient. Irrigate burns with large amounts of water or Milton's solution if available. Leave small blisters alone. Unroof large blisters (remove the loose overlying skin) and irrigate frequently with water and soap. Antihistamines may be useful to control itch. Eyes should be irrigated with copious amounts of saline initially then daily irrigations.

Where available antibiotic eye drops should be used. Upper airway symptoms may respond to steam inhalation or cough suppressants. In the case of Lewisite exposure there is an antidote (BAL aka Dimercarprol) for systemic exposure. For mustard gas there is a specific decontamination powder but it is not readily available.

Chapter 14 Wound Closure and Suturing

Contents

Stitching up gaping cuts in the bush with your darning needle and fishing line are the stuff great stories are made of. Certainly this can be effective but like anything it carries a risk if not done properly; poor healing, infection, and reactions to the suture material. Many wounds that we currently suture will heal very well without any intervention, and suturing is mostly done to speed up wound healing and for cosmetic reasons. Before you perform any surgical procedure you need to weigh up the benefits vs. the risks; suturing is no different - first do no harm.

However, suturing isn't hard and only requires adherence to a few basic principles. We are not going to discuss actual techniques for suturing though. A number of the books listed in the reference section provide detailed instruction on suture techniques. An area which is poorly covered and where there is a great deal of inaccurate information is regarding suture materials and needles. In a pinch your fishing line and a normal sewing needle may be ok, but they are far from ideal. So if you are stocking up you need to understand what to buy and why.

The manufacturers of suture material have a wealth of material available on their websites:

Ethicon: http://www.jnjgateway.com/public/USENG/Ethicon_WCM_Feb2004.pdf

Basics:

Tensile strength is how long a suture can be relied on to hold tissues together. Absorption is how long it takes for the suture material to be absorbed by the body.

Sutures are classified as:

Absorbable   natural or synthetic

Or

Non-absorbable   natural or synthetic

And

Monofilaments – suture made of a single strand

Or

Braided – suture made of several filaments twisted together

Natural absorbable:

Contents

Surgical Gut: Collagen material derived from the submucosal layer of sheep or the serosal layer of cattle intestines. Almost pure collagen.

Absorbed by enzyme action. Several types:

Plain gut: Tensile strength for 5-7 days, absorption within 42 days. Used primarily for ligating blood vessels and closing the fat layer.

Chromic gut: Gut treated with chromium salts. Strength for 7-10 days and absorption within 70 days. Versatile material commonly used for closing bowel, uterus, and episiotomy/tear repairs; ok for skin but not first choice.

Natural Non-Absorbable:

Surgical Silk: Spun by the silk worm. Braided. Tensile strength for

up to one year. Causes a significant soft tissue reaction. Hold knots very well. No longer indicated for routine use. Much better products available

Surgical linen: Braided multifilament obtained from flax; not commonly used.

Stainless steel: commonly used either as staples for the skin, for wiring the sternum following cardiac surgery, or for tendon repairs

Synthetic Absorbable:

Most are synthetic protein polymers. Exact names vary with which company has produced them but each company has equivalent products.

Polydioxanone (PDS), Monocryl: Monofilament. 60-70 % strength at 1 week and 40-50% at 3 weeks; absorption takes 3-4 months. Useful for internal sutures and subcutaneous use.

Polyglactin 910 (Vicryl, Polysorb): Braided, 65% strength at 1 week. Absorption takes approximately 2 months. Very versatile suture, useful for most things: Skin, internal tissues, episiotomy/tear repairs.

Synthetic Non-absorbable :

Nylon/Polypropylene (Prolene): Monofilament; high tensile strength material; low tissue reaction. Ideal for skin closure.

Contents

Thread Size:

Sizes range from 11-0 to 7. i.e. 11-0, 3-0, 2-0, 1-0, 0, 1, 2, 3 7

- 1. is the smallest with increase in size to 7

Commonly 3-0 or 2-0 is used for the skin. If working on the face a slightly smaller thread such as 6-0 or 5-0 may be used. For connective tissue 0 or 1 is a common size. Strength increases with the increasing size of the thread. Tissues under more stress and tension require a stronger thread.

Needles:

Two basic shapes - Curved

- Straight

Most common : 3/8 to ½ circle curved needle Three main types of needles:

- o
  - Taper: Sharp point which tappers down to a circular needle. Most versatile general purpose needle
  - Cutting: Triangular-shaped needle point with a cutting edge on the inside curvature of the needle. This type works well on tough tissues. Not good for the amateur.
  - Reverse cutting: Triangular-shaped needle with the cutting edge on the outside curvature of the needle. Again, good on tougher tissues and easier to use than a cutting needle.

Suture Removal:

Most sutures can be removed after 5 or 6 days. If the area is under a lot of stress such as the abdominal wall or over a joint or active muscle then 7-10 days.

Alternative methods:

Staples: Staples can be used interchangeably with sutures for closing skin wounds. They are equally as effective and very easy to apply. Their main drawback is that from a cosmetic standpoint they are inferior to sutures. They are also very expensive. They come in several sizes ranging from 10 staples to 100. Brand names include 3M and the United States Suture Company (USSC).

Glue: Glue is useful for small, superficial skin lacerations; lacerations only partial thickness or just into the subcutaneous layer. When used correctly it provides equivalent tensile strength to sutures. It should not be used around the eyes or mouth, and it is less effective in hairy areas. There are several brands of glue available, i.e.

Histacryl and Dermabond. The issue of using Superglue is addressed in the Q&A section (Q.8)

Hair tying: Not perfect but has been successfully used for scalp lacerations. The wound should be cleaned, and hair along the edges of the wound formed into bundles, and then opposite bundles tied across the wound to bring the edges together. After 5-7 days the hair can be cut from the wound edges.

Alternative suture material: A number of materials can be substituted for commercial suture material in austere situation. Possible suture materials include – fishing and sewing nylon, dental floss, and cotton, and in an absolute worse case horse hair or home made "gut" sutures. The latter two should only be considered in an absolute worse case scenario. If you only have improvised suture material available

you should seriously consider if suturing is the right thing to do. Anything which is organic has a much greater chance of causing tissue irritation and infection.

Alternative needles: Consider small sail makers, glove makers or upholsters needles. In theory any sewing needle can be used – but curved ones are obviously easier to use.

Summary:

Our view is that the most versatile material is a synthetic absorbable suture like Vicryl (or an equivalent), in a variety of sizes with a 1/3 circle taper needle. If Vicryl is unobtainable or too expensive then we recommend stocking nylon and simple gut in a variety of sizes. We would not recommend silk except in the absence of any alternatives. It is also worth considering disposable staplers if your finances stretch to that. Please remember, if you don't know what you're doing you may well make it worse.

Chapter 15 Austere Dental Care

In an austere or survival situation the ability to provide even limited dental care will be an extremely valuable trade commodity – a licence to print money.

ontents

The educational resources for dental care by non-dentists are limited. "Where There Is No Dentist" by Murray Dickson (see references) is the best single book around. It is limited in the details of its coverage of dental anaesthesia and modern filling material, but, otherwise, is an excellent and easy to understand introduction to dental care.

There are several other good web-based resources:

Common Dental Emergencies: http://www.aafp.org/afp/20030201/511.html

Merck Manual Dental Emergencies:

http://www.merck.com/mrkshared/mmanual/section9/chapter107/107a.jsp

Like much in this book the following information is offered for interest only and is no substitute for professional dental care. Much of this information is useless without detailed anatomical knowledge and instruction in actual techniques. We are not trying to teach dentistry here but are providing an overview of what is possible in austere situation, and helping you focus your preparations, and further education.

The basics of dentistry can simplistically be broken down into 7 areas:

Preventive dentistry:

Like preventive medicine the importance of preventive dentistry cannot be over emphasised. Before finding yourself in an austere environment get in the habit of daily brushing, and flossing, and regular dental check-ups, and appropriate treatments. When access to regular dental care is no longer possible then continuing with daily flossing and brushing is vital. High sugar foods and drinks particularly between main meals should be discouraged. Brushing alone is insufficient – you must floss as well.

Scaling and Cleaning:

This is simply an extension of preventive dentistry. While regular cleaning and flossing will minimise and slow plaque build-up it will still occur. This takes the form of mineralised deposits at the edges of the teeth and the gums, and just below the gum margins. This material is difficult to remove with simple brushing.

Scaling is the process where this material is scraped off using a scaler or dental pick. It is usually a relatively straightforward process.

Dental Pain and Infection:

Contents

Dental Pain

Pulpitis – inflammation of the dental pulp = toothache

This pain is often referred to surrounding area or radiates to other teeth. It can be difficult for patient to ID the exact tooth which is originating the pain. The tooth is usually not sensitive to percussion or palpation but maybe sensitive to heat, cold, sweets.

Frequently there is obvious cause, e.g. a large cavity. Management is by symptom control with oral antiinflammatories, and pain medications, local nerve blocks, cold packs, saline gargles, and soft diet. This management is standard for a number of conditions and will be referred to as "standard dental first aid" in the rest of this chapter.

Periapical Inflammation – Inflammation, but not infection, at the apex (root base)

The involved tooth is usually is easily located. The tooth may protrude a bit and/or cause pain with chewing. Usually there is no obvious external swelling as is the usual case with infection. Management is as for pulpitis.

Aphthous Ulcers – Lesion on oral mucus membranes, cause unclear

There are often multiple ulcers lasting 7 – 15 days. May be triggered by trauma, stress. Management is with standard dental first aid. Topical steroids may shorten course of healing

Muscle Pain & Spasm – chewing muscle dysfunction due to teeth grinding, jaw clenching, heavy chewing, etc. Management by muscle rest, soft diet, antiinflammatories.

Other Causes

Infections (discussed below), facial nerve pain, herpes zoster, vascular pain-migraine, sinus pain, referred pain.

Infections:

Herpes Labialis (viral) = cold sores on lips, tongue, gingiva, palate

Often triggered by sunburn, stress, and trauma. The patient often has a "prodrome" or tingle/pain before lesion presents. Management is by oral antiinflammatories, and pain medications, soft diet. Antivirals such as Acyclovir 200 mg 5x/day can shorten course. Mouth rinse of equal parts Maalox, Benadryl liquid, and Viscous Lidocaine may be soothing, swish & spit out, use every 2 hours as needed.

Oral Candidiasis (fungal) = Thrush; caused by overgrowth of yeast normally found in the mouth

Contents

Often seen in the very ill, immunocompromised, or those on/recently taking antibiotics. It looks like white spots or patches throughout mouth, may have a "cottage cheese" appearance, can be rubbed off, the patient's mouth and throat often very sore & red. It is managed by eliminating source of re-infection (toothbrushes washed in boiling water & air dried, etc.) and antifungal medicines. Topical antifungals like Nystatin Swish & Spit 5x/day or Mycelex Troche 4x/day. A good substitute is any sort of vaginal yeast cream rubbed into mouth & gums 4x/day. Oral antifungals like Diflucan 100 mg tablets 2x/day until it clears can also be used

Bacterial Infections

Many different organisms can cause infections often mixed aerobic and anaerobic bugs that are normally in the oral cavity. Infections can be life threatening if the infection spreads to deep tissues or into the brain. Fever, local swelling, and lymph node swelling is common.

Apical Abscess/Cellulitis – Infection of the pulp extending down to the bone & gum. The gum and tooth base appear normal. This is an infection at the very apex of the roots that has eaten through the thin bone of the jaw. Notable for fever, pain, often an abscess/pus pocket, or swelling will form where the gum tissue joins the lip, no sensitivity to heat or cold. Management is by incision & drainage through the gum to the level of the bone. A small improvised drain such as a portion of rubber band or cotton wick, will speed healing – remove when no longer draining. Dental first aid treatment should be applied. Antibiotics may be required, see discussion below. Tooth extraction is indicated if not resolving despite treatment.

Gingival/Periodontal Abscess – Infection between the gum and the tooth. The abscess is usually on the cheek side. The tooth is usually sensitive to percussion but not heat or cold. Manage with incision & drainage and dental first aid. Antibiotics are usually not necessary.

Pericoronitis – Infection of the gum overlying a partially erupted tooth such as a wisdom tooth. It often occurs in the back reaches of the mouth. It can mimic a peritonsillar abscess or pharyngitis although there usually is no drainage or purulence with this. Muscle spasm in the chewing muscles is common also. It is managed by cleaning out between the tooth & gum and dental first aid measures. Antibiotics are usually not necessary. At times removal of some of the redundant gum tissue may be helpful.

Deep Tissue/Fascia Infections – Any intraoral infection can spread quickly through the relatively loose tissue planes to other areas in the neck causing tissue breakdown, bleeding, and obstruction of the posterior pharynx and airway.

Immediate incision & drainage is required along with aggressive antibiotic therapy and supportive care. This is a potentially life-threatening emergency, and you should try to get help if you possibly can.

When to use antibiotics:

Dental abscesses are best treated by drainage of any collection present. Antibiotics should be used in patients who are systemically unwell – high temperatures, chills or shakes, nausea, vomiting, or gross local swelling.

Penicillin 500 mg 4x/day or Erythromycin 500 mg 3x/day are usually acceptable antibiotics. Broader spectrum drugs can also be used. For patients who are very unwell the addition of the drug metronidazole 400 mg 3 times daily or Tinidazole 2 gm once daily to cover anaerobic bacteria may be helpful.

Drilling and Filling:

Cavities on teeth cause pain either because they allow infection into the inside of the tooth or they expose nerve endings in the pulp of the tooth which is stimulated by exposure to temperature extremes or extreme sweetness.

It is very straightforward to provide a temporary filling which covers the hole and protects the exposed nerve endings. This can be done with a number of temporary filling materials available on the market. IRM – a mixture of zinc oxide and eugenol [oil of cloves] is considered one of the best commercial preparations which you can prepare yourself from the two ingredients. It is prepared by forming it into a firm paste and "puttying" over the cavity with it. These agents are, however, temporary.

Permanent fillings are more complicated. They have traditionally required the cavity to be opened up (frequently the hole on the surface of the tooth is small, with a much larger decayed area below), the decayed material removed, then the cavity sealed with a permanent filling agent. The cavity is opened up and cleaned with a dental drill.

It is unlikely that you will have access to a dental drill and associated permanent filling agents. However, the World Health Organization has developed a process known as Atraumatic Restorative Treatment (ART) technique. The ART technique involves caries removal and tooth filling (or restoration to use the correct term) with adhesive filing materials using hand instruments only, no drills. It has been specifically designed to be delivered by people with limited experience in dental procedures and often provided under primitive field conditions. This makes it ideal for a survival or austere situation. This is a step beyond temporary fillings and while they may not last a lifetime they may last many years. The equipment to perform ART

should be seriously considered as part of your preparations. An overview of the process and more detailed information is described at:

Atraumatic Restorative Techniques Step By Step .pdf:

http://216.26.160.105/conf/hrsa04/presentations/Bolin_3.pdf

ART Manual: http://www.dhin.nt/art_manual main.htm

The process requires some basic equipment:

A glass ionomer: Fuji IX GP Glass Ionomer is one example.

Contents

Cotton pledgets + absorptive gauze: The work area needs to be kept dry from saliva.

Mouth mirror: This is used to reflect light onto the field of operation, to view the cavity indirectly, and to retract the cheek or tongue as necessary

Tweezers: This instrument is used for carrying cotton wool rolls, cotton wool pellets, wedges, and articulation papers from the tray to the mouth and back.

Explorer: This instrument is used to identify where soft carious dentine is present. It should not be used to poke into very small carious lesions. This may destroy the tooth surface and the caries arrestment process. It should also not be used for probing into deep cavities where doing so might damage or expose the pulp.

Dental Hatchet: This instrument is used for further widening the entrance to the cavity thus creating better access for the excavator, and for slicing away thin unsupported carious enamel left after carious dentine has been removed.

Spoon Excavator: This instrument is used for removing soft carious dentine. There are 3 sizes:

- small: diameter of approximately 1.0 mm
- medium: diameter of approximately 1.2 mm
- large: diameter of approximately 1.4 mm

Mixing block and spatula: These are necessary for mixing glass ionomer. These items are included with the Fuji IX pack.

Applier/Carver: This double-ended instrument has 2 functions: The blunt end is used for inserting the premixed glass ionomer into the cleaned cavity and into pits and fissures. The sharp end is designed to remove excess restorative material and to shape the glass ionomer.

These instruments can be viewed at: http://www.gcasia.info/content_art_instrument.html

This process results in filings which are not as robust as those done with the conventional techniques, and some parts of some teeth are impossible to access without the assistance of a dental drill. Also the materials do not cope well on load bearing teeth surfaces but it does provide an alternative to extraction and may work well for years.

If you are planning for a longer-term scenario in a truly austere situation it is worth looking at dental history for some options for drilling and filling.

Contents

The process of drilling involves a small rapidly turning bit cutting through overlying bone to open up a cavity. Different drill bits or other handheld instruments are then used to remove the decay. Drilling is painful, and the more slowly the drill turns the more painful it is. This is overcome with modern high-speed pneumatic dental drills with thousands of revolutions per minute (rpm). Local anaesthesia can be used and often is; with a modern drill it frequently isn't required. However with a slow improvised drill it will be very painful without local anaesthesia. In improvising a dental drill you should look back at the first dental drills from several hundred years ago. The basic concept was using a foot pedal (like an old sewing machine or spinning wheel) or bicycle to generate rpms on a wheel – the faster the better. This rotational speed then needs to be transferred to the hand piece with the drill bit attached. This can be relatively easily accomplished with a series of pulleys.

Improvising the drill bit is potentially more di cult but in theory any small tapered metal tip (the head of a very small nail or tack) could be suitable.

Once you have overcome the problem of a dental drill you have the problem of finding a suitable restorative product. Gold is probably your best option. The use of gold film fillings has slowly faded over the last 20 years as better substances which are easier to place have become available. The basic technique is that the tooth is drilled, the cavity cleaned, a small ball of very thin gold film is placed in the defect to be filled, and it is slowly tapped and moulded into place with a dental pick. The description makes it sound easy – it isn't, and learning the technique has psychologically scarred many a dentist.

Aside from gold film there is no permanent dental filling which can be easily manufactured; in an austere situation extraction of the tooth may be the best option.

Dental Trauma:

Related Head & Neck Injury – Any blow or force strong enough to cause dental injury is potentially severe enough to produce injury to the head, other facial structures, and/or neck. Consider the possibility of cervical spinal injury, and evaluate ABC's (Airway, Breathing, Circulation) before getting focused or distracted by the dental injury.

Crown Chip – Small lines or "crazing" in the enamel. These are harmless.

Simple Crown +/- Root Fracture – The tooth is fractured but no pulp is exposed.

This is usually not a problem although sometimes it can be cold sensitive. Smooth rough edges with a nail file and remove small fragments. If the tooth is especially sensitive Eugenol (clove oil) or IRM can be used as a topical covering plus dental first aid measures.

Contents

Complicated Crown +/- Root Fracture – The pulp is exposed but the root is intact. Remove any fragments/pieces. Flush the area thoroughly with saline. If the pulp has been exposed for more than 24 hours remove about 2 mm of the pulp tissue. Seal the exposed pulp with Dycal, IRM, Glass Ionomer, or wax. Try to construct a smooth surface that will not irritate surrounding tissue or trap food particles, dental first aid measures. Tooth extraction is an option if pain is not manageable or infection develops.

Root Fracture – A fracture below the gum line involving one or more roots. May be difficult to distinguish between this and luxation of the entire tooth (see below).

Remove all fragments. If the entire crown is broken away do not attempt to extract the roots and apex. Reposition the tooth and stabilize by splinting with wire & brace bar, adhesive ribbon, or similar technique (discussed below). It takes a minimum of three months for the bone to heal. If necessary seal any exposed pulp tissue as above. Plus dental first aid measures. Tooth extraction is an option if pain is not manageable or infection develops.

Subluxation & Concussion – The tooth remains in normal position. In subluxation the tooth is abnormally loose due to damage of the periodontal ligament and gingiva; in concussion the tooth is only tender not loose. Avoid chewing on the loose tooth.

Excessively loose teeth may need to be splinted. Plus dental first aid measures.

Lateral Luxation – The tooth is intact but the root has been displaced breaking the surrounding bone. Often there is a bulge of the gum tissue indicating where the root has been pushed out of the socket. There may be a high metallic ring on percussion. Place the tooth back into normal position by pushing the root back into the socket while pulling out on the distal portion in a "teeter-totter" motion. Splint the tooth if needed plus dental first aid measures. Tooth extraction may be required if pain is not manageable or infection develops.

Intrusion – The tooth is driven deeper into the socket. Use dental first aid measures. Long-term tooth survival is poor. Tooth extraction if pain is not manageable or infection develops.

Extrusion – The tooth is partially pulled down out of the socket. The tooth is gently replaced into the socket and splinted if needed. Have the patient bite down gently to ensure that the tooth is all the way back in. Plus dental first aid measures. Tooth extraction if pain is not manageable or infection develops.

Tooth Loss – The tooth is knocked completely from the socket. Do not touch the root segment, or scrub the tooth, or the socket. Rinse the tooth with saline until clean, as well as the socket. Replace as soon as possible into the socket and splint. If immediate replacement is not available, store the tooth in saline, milk, or saliva. Implantation after 24 hours has little chance of success. Splint in place plus dental first aid therapy.

Segment/Jaw Fracture – Fracture of the bony structure of the jaw with 2 or more teeth involved. The teeth move independently of each other. Replace as with a subluxation and splint in place for 6 weeks.

Injuries To Primary "Baby" Teeth – Normally these are not repaired unless needed for comfort care of the patient. Plus dental first aid measures. Tooth extraction if pain is not manageable or infection develops.

Soft Tissue Injuries – The tongue, gums, and oral mucus membranes are often injured at the same time as the teeth. The excellent blood supply promotes rapid healing, and infection is rare. Clean and thoroughly irrigate the wound with saline. Laceration of ducts and glands can be di cult to repair and may cause ongoing problems – think in 3D when looking at facial injuries and considering what may have been injured. Close the tissue, preferably with dissolving sutures, as soon as possible. If unable to close the tissue within 12 hours, wait, and then close after 5 days when the wound bacteria counts have dramatically lowered. Ensure that the vermilion border of the lip is carefully repaired. For wounds all the way through the cheek close the mucus membrane from the inside then close the muscle and skin from the outside in standard fashion. Use 2 sets of instruments if possible to minimize contamination of the wound with oral flora. Use standard dental first aid measures.

An overview of serious facial trauma is given in this presentation:

http://www.brooks.af.mil/dis/DOWNLOAD/maxillofacialtrauma.ppt

Intra-oral splinting:

Splinting can be required for tooth dislocations and fractures, and fractures of the mandible (the lower jaw bone).

There are several techniques to temporarily splint a tooth dislocation or fracture.

Option 1. Wire suture material (or reasonably heavy gauge fuse wire) can be used to splint the tooth. The wire is glued to the affected tooth and to the neighboring teeth to provide stability.

Option 2. Cotton fibers can be mixed in with temporary filling mix and the resultant fibrous mix can be molded to make a splint between the injured tooth and its healthy neighbors.

For mandibular fractures or multiple involved teeth then full wiring of the jaw may be required 4-6 weeks. The technique is relatively straight forward:

Using small lengths of wire suture (or fine fuse wire) make a small loop in the center of the piece of wire. Wrap the wire in a figure 8 pattern around two teeth, with the small loop facing outwards, over the gap between the two teeth. Repeat this top and bottom – in at least 3-4 positions – so you have the loops top and bottom-lining up.

- Wire each pair of loops (the top and bottom ones) together, so the jaw is unable to open.
- The patient will be on a liquid diet for the duration of the wiring.

Extractions:

Before antibiotics this was the main treatment for dental infections. An infection in the root of the tooth could only be treated by pulling the tooth and allowing it to drain.

The basic underlying principle of dental extractions is very simple: the tooth needs to be loosened from its attachments to the gum and jaw, and then the tooth is gently rocked backwards and forwards until loose enough to be removed. The key point is

the gentle rocking rather than attempting to simply pull the tooth out. However, the reality can be much more complicated.

Firstly like setting a bone the process is very painful. There are a number of very effective local anaesthetic blocks which are easily used.

Secondly it can be difficult to grasp the tooth without the proper instruments although not impossible. The minimum instruments required to safely extract a tooth include a Maxillary Universal Forceps (150), Mandibular Universal Forceps (151), and a periosteal elevator. That said it is possible to remove a tooth with any solid grasping instrument – such a pair of pliers – with the tips wrapped in gauze or in some other way padded – although this is not recommended.

Thirdly if the tooth's root(s) breaks (which is more likely with decayed teeth and if the operator is inexperienced) then it can be impossible to remove and the broken root fragment will act as a focus for further infection. "First do no harm"

Prosthetics

The ability to chew food is pretty fundamental to survival. In some primitive societies when you lost your teeth to chew with then by nature of their diet you died – potentially a problem again.

Your priority should be to prevent yourself or your families from getting to the point where you have no teeth. The only option you will have is making some form of dentures.

Contents

To manufacture dentures will require significant effort and improvisation skills. Historically porcelain was used to manufacture dentures until the end of the 18th century. Recipes for porcelain were considered state secretes in some countries. Porcelain is glorified clay, and is moulded, and then fired to produce a very hard material – there is varying recipes – one recipe consists of one part each of silica, clay, and kaolin, 2 parts of Nepheline syenite, and a small amount of talc. There are many recipes. Before this time dentures had been manufactured out many substances including metal, bone, and animal and human teeth.

Dental kits and Instruments:

Another area around which there are frequent questions is dental instruments. Practically speaking you can remove a tooth with a pair of electrical pliers. However, if at all possible you should invest in some decent dental instruments. The instrument numbers are considered standard numbers but many companies have their own numbers or variations so check if you are unsure.

Level 1: Minimum Kit

This is the bare minimum that should be available. Note that all of this is obtainable at Wal-Mart, from many pharmacies, or similar stores. Often the majority of the components are sold as a "dental first aid kit".

Level 2: Basic Dental Kit

This is the minimum needed for basic dental work: temporary fillings and extractions. Where possible purchase supplies of high quality, they are reusable and will last for many years with proper care. Pretty much everything here is required for the kit as whole to be of value. The dental instruments are available from most medical instrument suppliers.

Level 3: Advanced Dental Surgery Kit

This is the advanced kit designed for those with some dental training and can do most needed dental work including fillings and extractions. Note that this kit builds on the basic dental kit and items can be added one at a time starting with the Flag or Cryer elevators, and Fuji IX ionomer cement, and building it up as skills and finance permit.

Note: Extractors 53R & 53L are mirror images of each other if you get the model with the straight handle. If you are nimble with your weak hand and can change sides on the patient you can get by with one or the other of the pair and save money and weight.

Note: Forceps # 18, 73, 75, 87, 201, and deep root elevators are of value also if you want to be really complete.

Table Basic dental kit

1

Contents

Contents

1

1

1

1

Dental mirror

Explorer/probe double end #5 Angle point tweezers

Excavator, double-end #38/39 or 38/40 Plugger/filler, double-end #1/2 or 1/3 or similar Elevator #301

Extraction forceps #150 universal upper

Extraction forceps #150 universal lower (can use #75 also)

Eugenol (oil of cloves) and zinc oxide powder, or IRM permanent filling material Cavity temporary filling material

Scalpel handle and #11 & #15 blades Needle driver, 4-5"

Scissors, Iris, curved Copalite cavity varnish

Sutures; 4-0 or 5-0; silk, or, Ethilon, and chromic, or Vicryl, cuticular needle 25 gauge stainless wire

Dental floss Baby teething gel Super Glue gel

Anaesthesia; lidocaine 1% or 2%; syringes; needles Irrigation syringe

Cotton balls & 4x4s

Table Advanced Dental kit

1

1

Contents

Contents

Dental mirror

Explorer/probe, double-ended #5 Angle point tweezers

Excavator, double-ended #38/39 or 38/40 Plugger/filler, double-ended #1/2 and 3/4 or similar Elevator #301

Elevator #34

Flag/Cryer elevators; 30 & 31 or 39 & 40 Extraction forceps #150 universal upper

Extraction forceps #151 universal lower (can use #75 also) Extraction forceps #23 universal large molar

Extraction forceps #17 lower anterior

Extraction forceps #18, or #53R, or 53L upper anterior, see note below Curette, Gracey scaler; 11-12

Curette, Gracey scaler; 5-6 or Ivory C-1 Bone rongeur

Bone rasp

Fuji IX glass ionomer ARM material

Eugenol (oil of cloves) and zinc oxide powder, or IRM semi-permanent filling material

Cavity temporary filling material Scalpel handle and #11 & #15 blades Needle driver, 4-5"

Scissors, Iris, curved Copalite cavity varnish

Sutures; 4-0 or 5-0; silk, or Ethilon, and chromic, or Vicryl; cuticular needle 25 gauge stainless wire

Reinforcement bars Dental floss

Contents

Baby teething gel Super Glue gel

Anaesthesia: lignocaine 1% or 2%; syringes; needles Irrigation syringe

Cotton balls & 4x4's

Chapter 16

Nursing care in an austere environment

No treatise on the subject of austere medical care would be complete without addressing the issue of the provision of nursing care. This includes both the short and long term as well as the more urgent aspects of immediate care. Proper nursing care can be as much a lifesaver as it is a source of comfort. Whether professionally trained or home-grown the person charged by circumstance or design with providing for the day-to-day care of others needs to be ready to address the ever-changing and continuing needs of their patients. There will also need to be an acceptance from family or group members of a more collective responsibility for caring for the sick and injured, and that delegating all of the care which a sick patient currently receives from trained nursing staff in modern hospital to one person isn't practical or desirable. Family and friends will need to take a much more active role in helping the "nurse" look after their patient - assisting with companionship, bathing, and feeding the

patient.

For our purposes "nursing" refers to a type of care, i.e. ongoing day-to-day care as opposed to an occupational calling. The person(s) providing this care may have formal training or not. The goal is to provide for the entire range of physical and emotional demands caused by the patient(s) illness or injury.

Nursing care begins where urgent or immediate care leaves off once the patient is stabilized and any imminent threats or disabilities are addressed. Because the subject of nursing care per se is so vast it is not the intent of the authors to provide a complete how-to. In keeping with the general philosophy of the book this section is meant to provide an introduction only highlighting some of the factors involved in providing austere nursing care.

You will need to be familiar with a large bag of tricks that will make recuperation not only more bearable but also more likely. Not everyone will survive despite your best efforts. Often whether or not someone recovers from a traumatic event or a significant illness depends on the care they receive beyond the emergent or acute phases. Without excellent nursing care a person may survive and also recover nearly fully intact from a fractured femur, for instance, only to succumb weeks later to the effects of being kept bedfast. Blood clots in the lower legs caused by inactivity, infected bedsores that result from laying on their back for too long, or even pneumonia resulting from the use of a simple anaesthetic agent such as ether, may claim them long after the fracture has been set and the road to recovery is being well travelled. Simple nursing measures can go a long ways towards preventing any of these from occurring, or addressing them if they should.

On a more everyday basis there are also simple considerations to make austere nursing practical: how to properly assess a temperature using an old-fashioned mercury thermometer, how to administer a proper injection, reducing fever with

simple measures that do not include medications, and ensuring proper nutritional support.

Defining austere nursing practice

Elsewhere in this work we address the various aspects of emergent care when "regular" health care is not available, a la' where there is no doctor/clinic/emergency facility. This section will concentrate on the lack of a hospital or other facility providing the follow on care.

Austere nursing care is "the provision of ongoing treatment over a period of days, weeks or longer, using limited resources, little or no outside support and in the absence of a working modern medical care system". The role of the austere care nurse differs greatly from that of the modern "traditional" nurse. They must be adept at improvisation. They may be home trained or educated using a village health care worker model, or merely thrust into the role without any training beyond life experience. Even if educated in the traditional model of nursing by way of a college, university or hospital-based program one may find themselves thrust by circumstance or design into a role for which all your education and experience have failed to prepare you.

You may have to be your own lab technician, physical therapist, nutritionist and beyond. You may have the luxury of working with others or find yourself practicing completely independent of all outside assistance. Protocols and treatment regimens may have to be formulated on the fly depending on available resources and working conditions. Whatever your background you may be expected to provide continuous, ongoing care lasting anywhere from days to weeks, to months or in a very few cases perhaps years. In that respect the care provided is no different from the traditionally accepted nursing model of the day-to-day caregiver.

Successful practice of austere nursing may require you to assess, diagnose and treat based upon your own assessments absent the assistance of others educated beyond a basic nursing level. You may find yourself making decisions about what antibiotics to use, whether to close a wound or leave it open to heal by granulation, how to best address the nutritional requirements of your patient(s) and how to best ration scarce resources. In the end the ultimate responsibility may be yours alone to bear. The line between nursing care and medical care is a thin one and frequently crossed. Much of what is discussed in other chapters is relevant to nursing care and visa versa.

Remember this: by virtue of the circumstances under which you will be providing austere nursing care your decisions must be based upon what is in your patient's best interests and not governed by medical-legal considerations. If your world were in proper working order there would be little call for austere practices to begin with.

There will be no such thing as scheduled shifts, resupply a phone call or fax message away, and possibly no physician or other higher medical authority within travelling distance or in communication. Where regulation leaves off common sense and ethical considerations have to take over.

Developing the Proper Mindset

The first step in the process of adapting to the austere environment is developing the proper mindset. As stated above the rules by which modern medical care is provided have little or no application here. In an austere environment you will find that:

The system has broken down entirely either on a local scale or across the board.

The system doesn't apply, such as in backcountry areas of third world, and even some first world nations (examples of the latter: the Alaskan bush country, the Hudson Bay region of Canada, or the Australian Outback).

Occasionally circumstance prevents communication with the proper authority either due to physical difficulty or because of severe time constraints. Examples would include:

Lack of phone lines, radio-signal dead areas due to terrain or distance, and a lack of all-weather roads, or roadways blocked by physical obstacles (flooded rivers, mudslides, avalanche, and deep snow).

The time spent attempting to communicate with the proper authorities would endanger your patient.

Assuming one is trained, licensed, and authorized to practice as a nurse or other appropriate health care provider they will have to fall back upon the premise of what any reasonably competent person with equivalent skills and training would do given the same set of circumstances. A modern example would be nurses and other caregivers responding to the World Trade Centre crashes or the Asian tsunami.

Emergent and on-going care was provided in both situations without benefit of prior authorization or proper tools, making do with what was available based upon the assessed needs of those requiring care and the given environments.

In the absence of formal training a prudent person will identify their skills and the resources available and act within those boundaries. There is a wealth of information contained within the pages of this book that will set you well on your way to providing quality care under difficult circumstances. The overriding premise here is first to do no harm. Tightly linked with that premise is actually knowing what may legitimately constitute harm to begin with. The perceived benefits must outweigh the likely risks.

Use of this book does not constitute a license to practice medicine. Whatever the situation may be, you are morally if not legally bound to operate within the generally accepted standards of the ethical provision of care that aids in the recovery or comfort of your patient(s) without causing detriment by way of deliberate omission or a willful act of harm.

Hotel Care

This is an odd section title but it accurately describes an extremely important basic nursing function. It mirrors the fundamentals of what is required for survival – food/ warmth (shelter)/water/clothing – except when you are looking after patients you must provide these essentials for them. Absent imminent threat these are the most basic of all nursing care functions.

Water

Water is second only to air as being important to life. A person may survive weeks with no food but as little as 72 hours with no water. Ensuring adequate hydration is a significant part of basic nursing care. Lack of proper hydration may lead to prolonged healing, decreased ability to fight infection, altered levels of awareness, improper waste elimination, and in severe cases organ failure and eventual death.

Other than being taken by mouth water can be introduced rectally (proctoclysis) as detailed elsewhere in this book, and of course by the familiar intravenous route if properly prepared IV fluids are available.

Food

Patients may require varying diets that may differ significantly from what they are used to. For something as simple as a tooth extraction a diet of soft breads, ground meats and mashed vegetables may all they can tolerate due to difficulties chewing. Two recommended books that include dietary information are War Surgery Field Manual and Where There Is No Doctor. (See reference section for further details).

Warmth

The old adage about treating for shock by keeping a person warm has more than a ring of truth. Not only shock but also any number of ailments as well as injuries may cause a person to lose body heat. This is in addition to the issue of comfort. Besides covering them with warm blankets think in terms of warming the bed itself. Try a hot water bottle, a heated brick, or an old-fashioned bed warmer. All have been used for hundreds of years with good results. In the austere environment looking to the past for answers may provide answers to issues that otherwise seem insurmountable.

Linen

Clean linen and lots of it is one of the keys to providing good nursing care – sheets, blankets, washing cloths and towels. Until you have actually provided nursing care to a person it is hard to believe how much linen you can go through in a day. You should give some thought to how you will wash large amounts of linen possibly without access to electricity.

Recovery Care

Once a traumatic or medical situation is addressed in the immediate term we move on to the recovery, or subacute care, phase. During this period we will be concerned with addressing the continuing problems created by the illness or injury. Assuming that we will eventually have access to outside assistance our job of providing for such cases is simply a matter of ensuring that recovery continues or that the patient's condition at least remains stable. If there is no outside assistance likely in the foreseeable future

our task is then to ensure the patient's eventual recovery to their former state of health.

For most people this phase will be the most-time consuming. The patient may be suffering the after-effects of an acute illness, or require regular care for healing wounds and/or acute injury. In either situation their care is likely to require regular assessment of vital signs, elimination, pain, and overall function.

During this phase of care you may reasonably be expected to administer medications on an ongoing basis, perhaps change dressings and apply various treatments intended to promote healing of wounds and/or injuries, provide some or all of your patient's basic needs (reference Hotel Care above). You will need the use of various tools that make this phase of care practical, and to know the tricks that make such care practical as far as time and effort.

Care Planning

Just as important is taking time to step back and assess the overall situation and devise a plan of care to guide your efforts. This is not as complicated as it sounds. In the hospital and long-term care environments nurses develop what are routinely called "care plans." These are detailed plans of care that are intended to be unique to each patient's needs, and tend to be as much centered on medical-legal considerations as actual necessary care issues. For our purposes we need only to have a basic plan in place that is intended to ensure that the major aspects of required care are not overlooked.

A simplified care plan might take the following form if written out: Vital Signs: Check every 6 hours and record

Nutrition: Soft foods high in protein, 5 small meals per day totalling approximately 1,800 calories, snacks in evening as appropriate

Positioning: Elevate broken leg on pillows to keep above heart level. Use propping pillows to position from side to side at regular intervals

Elimination: Check every 2 hours to see if they need the bedpan or urinal Pain: Assess pain level every 3-4 hours and give medication as needed

Contents

Medication: administer scheduled medication at 8:00 AM, 4:00 PM and Midnight

For an uncomplicated case of flu with only one caregiver care a written plan, as simple as it is, may not be needed. Simply establish a routine and follow it. If more than one patient is involved or there is more than one nursing care provider having a simple written plan of action can eliminate potential mistakes and miscommunication such as administering medication twice or overlooking a significant change in the vital signs.

Basic Nursing/Patient Care Tools

As with any other endeavor you will require certain tools of the trade. Tools to assess vital signs, to address bodily functions, to make administration of medications possible, and to make ongoing care practical. Aside from obviously disposable items such as bandages and dressings durable goods are the most practical for situations where resupply intervals may be few and far between, or even non-existent. Glass and stainless steel are two of your best friends in such situations. If planning on providing ongoing patient cares look for equipment that can be found in durable forms.

You will need tools that measure blood pressure, pulse rate, weight, fluid volume, and size (length, circumference, and diameter), and temperature. Examples of such tools would be:

Blood pressure cuff: Mercury column, aneroid (dial-type) gauge, or an electronic device such as a wrist or self-inflating arm cuff. Mercury column devices maintain calibration longer than other types and can be used to calibrate aneroid gauges, which are more portable. Electronic devices are great timesavers but are more prone to loss of calibration and inaccuracy as batteries are depleted.

Watch or clock: In order to obtain accurate pulse and breathing rates you need a digital display with a seconds' count, or a sweep-hand that is marked in seconds as well as minutes.

Graduates and other fluid measuring devices: Used to accurately measure urine output and also fluid intake. Common kitchen measuring devices with a capacity of 32 oz (1 liter) or greater will work well. A see-through container with measurement markings will make the task much easier. This may see a lot of use so durability is preferred.

Stethoscope: Assessing lung and bowel sounds is a basic part of nursing care. You are checking for abnormal sounds in the lungs, and the presence or absence of sounds in the abdominal area. A good quality single-head stethoscope with spare diaphragms is a must-have piece of equipment.

Scale: The type of scale isn't as important as the fact that whatever device is used measures the same way each time. The actual scale can be electronic, mechanical, or improvised such as a balance beam and counterweights of known measurement. Even

Contents

water displacement can be used so long as you have a means of measuring the volume accurately since water has a known weight per volume.

Fabric Tape Measure: Wounds may need to be measured to gauge healing progress. Edema (swelling) needs to be measured to determine if treatments are effective.

Bandages may need to be measured for fit. A measuring device that will wrap around an extremity is more practical than a rigid ruler.

Thermometers: Thermometers have a variety of uses in the austere environment. Fever charting can confirm a diagnosis or help you differentiate between diseases. Knowing core temperatures is important in managing environmental emergencies. Body temperature monitoring also has other applications.

Determining morning basal temperatures (by taking the temperature first thing in the morning before getting out of bed or moving around much) is important in identifying and managing certain chronic conditions. For instance, if you have someone in your group who is hypothyroid (common today because hyperthyroidism is treated by destruction of the thyroid), and are using the expedient management technique of giving them a half a sheep's thyroid every day or two, watching the basal temperature for spikes is a good way to know when to skip a dose or, conversely, a dip indicates a need for a bit extra. Basal temperatures are also used for other purposes, such as determining the expected time of ovulation for women desired to become pregnant.

All of this means that you should include at least one, and preferably several, thermometers in your kit. Clinical thermometers used to be all one of one basic kind - the mercury thermometer - but today you have a variety of options, including electronic thermometers, electronic tympanic membrane thermometers, and single use (disposable) thermometers. All have advantages and disadvantages. If you expect to be in the austere environment for an extended period without resupply you should choose the old-fashioned mercury thermometer, since they will keep working forever

–if- you don't break them. However, you should also count on breaking them, and may want to consider doubling or even tripling the number of thermometers you purchase above the recommended number to help guard against this. Electronic thermometers have the advantages of speed and accuracy (digital basal thermometers are available with readouts to 1/100th of a degree, for instance), but you will need batteries or some other means of powering them (use at least a rinse followed

by a dry wipe followed by an alcohol pad wipe to clean them between uses if you don't have the sheaths). Electronic thermometers may also be usable over wider ranges than conventional thermometers. Electronic tympanic membrane thermometers (which let you read temperature from the ear) make it easy to avoid cross-infection, but again, they need a power supply. Disposables are great for preventing cross-infection, but when they're gone, they're gone.

Classes of specialty clinical thermometers

Contents

Standard thermometers - thermometers with a temperature range usually limited to about 35-42 degrees (94-108 degrees F).

Basal thermometers are thermometers designed to be read to at least 1/20th of a degree (1/10th of a Fahrenheit degree), rather than the 1/10th degree (2/10th of a Fahrenheit degree) of most standard mercury thermometers.

Hypothermia thermometers are thermometers that allow the reading of temperatures lower than standard thermometers, usually having ranges that extend down to 30 degrees (86 degrees F) or lower.

Hyperthermia thermometers are thermometers that allow the reading

of higher than normal temperatures to more accuracy than standard thermometers.

Purchase recommendations: *For each ten people have at least two standard thermometers, one basal thermometer, and one hypothermia thermometer.*

Hyperthermia thermometers should be purchased at the rate of one to every twenty people if you expect to see heat injuries commonly, otherwise, a normal clinical thermometer will usually suffice.

Rectal versus oral versus universal tips - get universal tips (midway between oral and rectal, and they can be used for either in a pinch) for the clinical and basal

thermometers, rectal for the hypothermia and hyperthermia thermometers.

Then there are the simple but easily overlooked tools that make ongoing care not only practical but less strenuous and safer for both patient and caregiver.

Bandage Scissors: Designed to cut away bandages next to the body without poking holes in your patient. They combine safety with practicality.

Permanent Marker: To write on dates or times on dressings to know when they were last changed if there is more than one caregiver. Also used to mark disposable items that should not be shared between patients. Also used to mark skin (it wears off with repeated washing and normal skin replacement).

Transfer Belt: Known by various names such as walking belt, safety belt, gait belt, etc. The commercial version is a 3" wide sturdy fabric strap that is easily buckled around the patient so the caregiver can assist them with standing up, transferring, or walking. It can also be fashioned from a pair of sturdy pants suspenders or an ordinary (wide) clothing belt. It provides a handle for the caregiver to grab on to by placing it around the middle (lower stomach area) of the patient and holding onto the rear of the belt.

Contents

Bedside Table: As simple as it seems having someplace to set things while providing care is extremely important. It isn't always practical to reach into your pocket for everything and setting tools, dressings, etc. on the bed itself may be asking to have them contaminated or kicked off.

Clothing Protectors: Another simple yet important item that can be fashioned readily from any soft or fluid resistant material. Intended to catch spills while eating/feeding and protect the patient while washing hair or performing treatments. They may tie behind the neck or have a wrap-around collar that fastens with Velcro. By protecting from spills they also save a lot of time by guarding against the necessity of clothing and bed linen changes.

Flashlight: This serves a dual role as both as assessment tool for the eyes, ears, nose and mouth, and the means to check a patient at night without awakening them with overhead lighting. Room lighting is not always adequate to view whatever may need to be seen.

Gowns: Caring for people may routinely require exposing differing areas of their body for washing, administering medications, changing dressings and bandages or measuring vital signs. Having to undress a person each time is time-consuming and impractical as well as potentially painful. Modesty dictates that we be able to cover the patient when exposure is not otherwise needed. Open back gowns while the bane of hospitalized patients world-wide represent the most practical means of combining protection with accessibility when shirt and pant style clothing is not practical or possible, as when casts or external appliances interfere. Something as simple as a sheet cut poncho-style will work nicely as well.

Nail Clippers: Finger and toenails continue to grow even when we are ill. Vanity issues aside it may be necessary to trim nails to address issues of hygiene (germs love to hide under nails) and prevent inadvertent self-injury by a patient who may flail about with pain or fever delirium. Having properly designed and sized clippers for the fingers and toes makes this task much easier for all concerned.

Providing On-Going Care

Having identified our goals we can move on the issue of how we are to address them. There are several areas that need to be addressed as part of the entire care "package" or plan.

Databases:

Vital Signs

Having a database of vital signs is the key to recognizing abnormal vital signs later on. In an ideal situation you would have a record that details normal laying, sitting and standing blood pressures for your patient, as well as a resting pulse, and respirations, along with a temperature. Make sure to note whether the normal pulse is

Contents

regular and strong in quality and rhythm, or irregular, weak, or bounding (very strong). Illness and/or injury may cause these measurements to change drastically. Assessing vital signs is covered in more detail later in the Q and A section. For the moment we will concentrate on a few of the "whys."

Temperature

Temperatures can be used to monitor for the presence and progression of infections, adverse reactions to medications, and dehydration. Having a database of temperatures over time will allow you to gauge the effectiveness of antibiotics, for instance, or the onset of an infection. Similarly a person who is acutely dehydrated will see an increase in their temperature.

Pulse

Pulses may indicate a general state of health in the absence of illness or injury. A very rapid, thin pulse may indicate the presence of shock, whereas a slow pulse might signal that the patient is relaxed and relatively pain free. Since pulse rates vary widely amongst people the change in pulse rate and quality is more important than the rate itself. For example, for a person whose normal pulse rate at rest is 68 an increase of 20 per minute may indicate the presence of unaddressed pain.

Blood Pressure

Blood pressures are always obtained using a blood pressure cuff, either manually operated or electronic. Cuffs come in different sizes with a standard blood pressure cuff suitable for adolescents and adults. An upper arm larger than approximately 15 cm will require a larger cuff for an accurate reading or a false high will result.

Conversely an arm smaller than approximately 8 cm will require a smaller diameter cuff or a false low reading will result.

Breathing

Normal breathing rates for an adult range between 14 and 20 per minute, or one breathe every 3 – 4 seconds. During times of illness this may increase, with more than 30 breaths a minute considered very significant.

In addition to rate the apparent effort used to breath can also be indicative of distress or absence of same. In a healthy person breathing should come easily and gently.

Respiratory infections can cause labored breathing, evidenced by increased effort and rate. By tracking breathing rates and quality along with other vital signs it is possible to determine whether treatments are having a positive effect.

Other Data to Collect and Record

Bowel Movements

Contents

As we age our bowel movements tend to become less frequent. Normal for an infant is several loose stools each day. Adolescents and adults may have one per day. Older

adults may not have a proper bowel movement for several days without regular use of fiber in their diet and/or laxatives. As a rule a person should have one medium to large bowel movement at least every 3 days.

Urination

It is not necessary to record urine outputs for everyone but for some cases – especially burns - measuring output against fluids taken in (Intake and Output) is necessary to determine whether fluid balance is being maintained. A healthy adult can be expected to void (urinate) 1,500 ml or more per day. The effects of disease, loss of fluids through other sources such as perspiration, vomiting, bowel movements, etc may affect this somewhat but as a general rule plan on a measured output of one and a half litres. Anything less than half this amount may be indicative of kidney malfunction and is cause for serious concern.

For certain types of patients, such as burn cases or those with heart failure, matching Intake and Output (I & O) against daily weights can be critical to determine if an

output deficit is the result of retained fluids.

Weight

Weight by itself may mean little other than as a general indication of nutritional status but changes in weight can be significant in terms of indicating changes in the patient's condition. For instance fluid retention or loss can vary a person's weight by several pounds (2 – 3 kilograms) per day. Sudden fluid gain can precipitate heart failure, and also may indicate failing kidney function if present along with decreasing urine output. Sudden weight loss normally indicates a loss of fluids from the body, a very important consideration with large-scale burns where we want to achieve balance in the body's fluid load.

Bed Mobility

The ability to change positions in bed is often taken for granted by those not affected by illness or mobility problems. Pressure sores, which will be addressed later in this section, are one potential problem of immobility. Increased tendency towards pneumonia is another.

Lifting Frames

Contents

One device useful for caregiver and patient alike is the overhead lifting frame, or trapeze bar. This is an overhead frame that is firmly secured to the bed, wall, or floor. The traditional model uses a triangular handle secured to the bar or frame positioned overhead by means of sturdy strap, rope, or chain. The bar or strap is used by the patient who has the upper body strength to lift themselves off the bed, allowing for self or assisted repositioning, or for the caregiver to change the bed linens without the patient exiting the bed. It saves both time and physical stress and offers the bedfast patient a sense of self-reliance.

Side rails

As simple as the concept sounds having removable railings alongside the bed may be an important factor for both patient and caregiver. Besides preventing a weak or disoriented person from inadvertently rolling out of bed they can be used by the patient for repositioning by providing them with a handle to grab onto to pull or roll themselves. Modern hospital beds have fold-down rails but removable railings can be fashioned by fitting them with "legs" that attach to the bedside using screw clamps or other type of easily removable fastener. This will allow for a measure of safety while also allowing full access for bedding changes and transfers. In most cases half rails that protect the upper half of the bed are sufficient.

Positioning

Positioning can be defined as the art of arranging the patient properly to encourage maximum retention of function, comfort, and accessibility. As simple as it seems improper positioning can and does lead to breakdowns in skin integrity, loss of function of limbs, and prolonged recovery times.

Elevation

Elevating the head of the bed aids in breathing for some people, especially in instances of pneumonia, asthma, and emphysema, and can assist with keeping the airway clear. It is also more conducive to eating and taking liquids. Simple techniques for achieving this in a bed not otherwise designed for the head to be elevated are to use blocks under the legs at the head end, or to place blocks, pillows or other items under the upper portion of the mattress.

Positioning Pillows

To reduce any tendency towards pressure sores and to increase patient comfort it is common practice to alternate the way patients lay by positioning them first on their left side, then their back, and finally on the right side before starting over, with changes every 2-3 hours.

Pillows are used to prop the person who is otherwise unable to lay on one side unassisted. They are also used to elevate limbs to reduce edema (swelling) and to provide comfort. Some people may also breath better with two or even three pillows under their upper back and head.

Other Positioning Aids

Contents

Besides pillows, blanket rolls, and folded towels may be used. These can be used by placing them between the knees, for instance, of the person who finds having their legs in straight alignment with their body uncomfortable but as they lie on their side it's a more comfortable pose.

Personal Hygiene

Personal hygiene is another significant area of concern. The patient may be unable to reach their back, for instance, due to arthritis or injury to the arms, back, or shoulders. They may be unable to bend at the waist and thus unable to cleanse themselves below that point.

Make arrangements to provide for regular bed baths, to trim fingernails, wash hair, and provide for basic oral hygiene by brushing teeth and rinsing the mouth. Wiping the person daily with a damp cloth helps control the odour of perspiration with a complete bed bath every 3-4 days recommended for most people.

Bodily Functions

You will need to provide for your patient's elimination requirements: urine, feces, and perspiration (sweat). Don't forget also that since we may be dealing with illness emesis (vomiting) is also a potential problem that will need to be dealt with. This is dealt with more in depth in the Q and A section below.

Pain Assessment

Pain is a particularly subjective experience with no two people experiencing it quite the same way. Identical injuries may elicit differing responses in different people. One person may find the same pain tolerable that another finds excruciating. There is no definitive measure of pain, but there are a couple of useful tools that offer clues as to how much pain the person is experiencing.

Pain is often measured using a 0 – 10 scale, with 0 (zero) being the complete absence of pain and 10 (ten) being considered to be the worst pain the person has ever experienced or the worst pain they can imagine, often referred to as excruciating pain.

Another scale often used is the 5-point scale which is graded as follows: 1 – No pain

1. – Mild pain
2. – Moderate pain 4 - Severe pain

5 – Overwhelming pain (the worst the patient can imagine)

In general any perceived pain that the patient describes as 2 (two) or above is worthy of being addressed,beginning with simple pain measures or remedies and progressing as needed. Ideally we would relieve the pain entirely but the very nature of austere medicine dictates that we may have to settle for reducing the pain to a level that is

Contents

either tolerable for the patient or at least allows them to function.

Nutrition

As mentioned previously two books recommended in the References section offer information about nutritional support in the austere setting. There is a wealth of information available both on-line and in print regarding nutrition but a few general suggestions are offered here:

Trauma victims in general, and burn victims specifically, require significantly more protein on a daily basis than an otherwise healthy person. In the austere environment plant protein alone is likely to be insufficient to meet these needs. Animal protein (meat) will provide a better balance of the complex proteins needed to rebuild damaged muscle tissues.

Orthopedic patients may recover faster with the addition of calcium supplements to their diet. In addition to milk and other dairy foods OTC supplements such as calcium-based antacid tablets may be of benefit to rebuilding damaged bones.

Following invasive procedures that involve the abdomen in particular a clear liquid diet is preferred until the patient regains normal bowel function. Clear liquids consist of water, broth, gelatins (flavored or not), and tea (but not coffee). The general rule of thumb in determining what constitutes a clear liquid is the ability to see the bottom of the cup or glass through the contents.

Breathing Care

Patients with chest infections or chest injuries (who are prone to chest infections) may need some help with their breathing. The mainstay of treatment for difficulty with breathing is to treat the underlying problem and oxygen – this is unlikely to be available to you, so you need to consider alternatives to assist with optimizing breathing.

Positioning is very important. Lying flat is not good for breathing. Semi-sitting or sitting upright is probably the best position for the patient with breathing difficulty.

Fully inflating the lungs with each breath also improves breathing, opening the smaller airways, and helping the body clear out mucus. This can be achieved by alternating asking the patient to try and blow up a balloon or a similar activity with sucking in through a straw for several minutes each 3-4 times a day

Percussion and postural drainage has been used extensively to help drain respiratory secretions in chest infections. While traditionally done by a physical therapist (physiotherapist) or respiratory therapist, cystic fibrosis parents have been taught for years how to perform it on their children and it is very straightforward. It helps loosen mucus and purulent secretions, and helps them to be coughed up.

The following is a simple overview of the process. It should be done with a cupped hand rather than a flat hand:

Contents

- Position the patient on his/her side on a pillow.
- Tilt the patient's head downward with his/her bottom above the level of his/her head. The position can be varied with the patient lying on their front or back – the key point is the head down position.
- Gently tap your patient's side with a cupped hand just under the armpit and across back.
- Reverse sides and repeat until your patient is able to expel some mucus.

A more detailed description (especially of more accurate hand positions) can be found at: http://www.questdiagnostics.com/kbase/as/ug1720/how.htm

Simple devices that may assist with breathing care include steam and cool mist vaporizers. Steam vaporizers are easy to improvise with something as simple as a pan of clean water set to heat near the patient and some sort of containment – such as a plastic sheet, or even a cloth sheet if nothing else is available - used to hold the mist in proximity to the patient. Simple medications such as menthol or herbal remedies can be placed in a pan over the heating water. Using salt water in a concentration of approximately 1% will also help some in clearing mucous.

A simple alternative to lack of electricity to power a nebulizer machine is to use a common bicycle pump to provide an intermittent but effective source of pressurized air that will vaporize whatever suitable medication is used in the chamber. This method of powering a nebulizer is, however, time consuming, and labor intensive.

Emotional Care

Emotional care is called for any time a person is ill or injured. It may be as simple as a mother's soothing words to a child with a stomach ache, or as involved as deliberate emotional support for the person who has suffered a significant injury and is experiencing a depression as a result of their misfortune.

Be aware that people experiencing ongoing pain and/or disability may become short- tempered and irritable. This is usually an unconscious response on their part that improves with recovery or increased comfort. The caregiver needs to be understanding of this and separate a temporary condition from true personality traits.

Simple comfort measures, observance of modesty issues, and sometimes just providing an ear for the patient to express their concerns or frustrations to can go a long ways towards addressing these issues. The person who is the subject of your care is likely to feel vulnerable if not outright helpless. Anything that can be reasonably done to reduce these feelings will make the situation more tolerable for the nursing care provider and the patient alike.

Physical Activity

Contents

Physical activity is a key issue for everyone. As noted previously immobile limbs tend to contract due to lack of muscle use. Simple range of motion exercises can aid greatly in preventing this as well as other complications. The key is gentle exercise.

Limbs should be flexed and extended within the normal limits of the joints as practical. Fingers should be flexed as well as the wrists, elbows, and shoulders. For the lower extremities: The hips, knees, ankles, and the toes if practical.

The person whose care requires casting for a period of time will find that upon removal of the cast the immobilized limb will be very weak. Begin with simple stretching and bending several times a day as pain levels allow. Don't be discouraged when progress seems to be slow. Even a muscular individual will find full recovery easily could take weeks before they have their full strength and range of motion restored

Chronic Care

In a situation where eventual access to outside assistance is not foreseeable there may come a point where care converts from that aimed at recovery to simply providing on- going care for a chronic condition. Whereas in cases of recovery, or subacute, care we center our care around rebuilding the patient's health here we are concerned with maintaining a level of health when further recovery is not likely. This does not automatically imply that the person is an invalid but rather than their condition has stabilized ,and they have achieved as much healing as they are ever likely to absent a fully functional modern health care facility.

Some injuries or ailments simply cannot be fully recovered from under austere conditions, whereas others may require additional weeks or months of low-level care, such as recovery from a major long bone fracture or a spinal fracture that does not result in a functional deficit. The result may be the need for reduced but nevertheless continuing care requirements. The patient may be confined to the house due to impaired mobility for instance. Even when able to move about with a wheelchair they still run the risk of future impairments due to their lack of full mobility.

For our purposes we are assuming that the condition is such that the person will eventually recover to the point that they are able to assume responsibility for most of their own care. They may still require assistance with such activities as preparing food, bathing, and getting into and out of bed, but are able to feed themselves, and move about with the aid of assistive appliances (wheelchair, crutches, cane, etc). A person who is truly bedfast and totally dependant upon others for all of their activities of daily living (bathing, eating, elimination, dressing, etc) will not likely survive long, succumbing eventually to infection or the effects of chronic immobility. While we intend to do what we can within the means available to us we must also face the possibility that some people will die no matter how attentive to their care we are. In this respect austere nursing care is no different from that of the present day.

Following are a list of potential conditions which the prevention of tops the list of concerns.

Bedsores:

Contents

More properly termed pressure sores or decubitus ulcers. They result from the pressure caused by the body resting on the same point(s) without shifting the weight off of the point(s) of contact. They are common in people who use wheelchairs or who are bedridden even for relatively short periods of time such as following a surgery, or persons who are emaciated, paralysed, or who suffer from decreased sensation. Key areas prone to development of pressure sores include the hips, the points of hip to the rear (the ischium), the sacrum (base of the spine), heels, and the shoulder blades.

General precursors to bedsores can be easily identified:

Elderly

Bedfast or wheelchair-bound

Unable to move certain parts of the body without assistance due to injury, illness, or weakness

Incontinence of bladder or bowels: moisture next to the skin can cause breakdown over time

Fragile skin due to age, disease, or injury

Prevention is the key. Check daily for reddened areas that do not blanch (turn white when pressed), blisters, sores, or craters. Other useful measures include:

- Change position every two hours to relieve pressure.
- Use items that can help reduce pressure -- pillows, sheepskin, foam padding, or semi-firm air mattress (never allow the person's skin to lie directly on a vinyl mattress though. The sweat build-up will itself cause further problems).
- Eat healthy, well-balanced meals.
- Exercise daily including range-of-motion exercises for immobile patients.
- Keep skin clean and dry. Incontinent people need to take extra steps to limit moisture.
- Tincture of green soap is an older remedy used to toughen skin in order to make it less prone to breakdown. It is a combination of vegetable soap, lavender oil, glycerine, and ethyl alcohol that is biodegradable, mildly antiseptic, and good skin degreaser. It is used by applying it straight to the skin surface to be treated.

Bedsores are categorized by severity from Stage I (early indications) to Stage IV (worst):

Contents

Stage I: A reddened area on the skin that, when pressed, is "non-blanchable" (does not turn white). This indicates that a pressure ulcer is starting to develop.

Stage II: The skin blisters or forms an open sore. The area around the sore may be red and irritated.

Stage III: The skin breakdown now looks like a crater where there is damage to the tissue below the skin.

Stage IV: The pressure ulcer has become so deep that there is damage to the muscle and bone, and sometimes tendons and joints.

Once a bedsore has been identified continue with preventive measures described above and additional treatment should begin immediately to avoid further degradation of the tissue:

- Relieve pressure to the area using pillows, foam cushions, or sheepskin
- Moisture barrier ointments such as Calmoseptine will be of significant benefit for Stage I or II sores only. Coating the area with talcum powder or a similar product before applying the cream will allow it to be cleaned off easier and will also help dry the skin underneath of the barrier coating. Solid cooking shortening (Crisco) or even lard can be used in the absence of medical creams. Petroleum jelly, however, should NOT be used. The ointment or cream selected should be applied at least twice per day and perhaps as often as every 4-6 hours if the patient is frequently incontinent of urine.
- Improve nutrition. A good multi-vitamin at a minimum should be part of the care. Zinc supplements in particular are also very useful in preventing skin breakdowns.
- Keep the area clean and free of dead tissue. Use salt water to cleanse and gently remove dead tissue. Never massage the area though as it can damage the sensitive tissue underneath.

Deep Vein Thrombosis:

More commonly associated in the lay press with "economy class syndrome" from air travel, Deep vein thrombosis is a very common cause of death for bed bound patients. It occurs do primarily to prolonged immobility, and is worsened by conditions such as lower limb fractures, cancers, or a genetic predisposition to clotting.

Contents

The best treatment is prevention. Where possible even significantly unwell patients should be mobilized several times a day somehow – the benefits of bed rest need to be balanced against the risks of developing clots. Patients should not cross their legs in bed, and massage and stretching of the legs should be encouraged 3-4 times per day as a minimum. The best preventive treatment is daily injections of subcutaneous heparin

– but this won't be an option for many.

Contractures:

This refers to the tightening of the non-bony tissues of the muscles, skin, ligaments, or tendons. Unless promptly addressed the condition will become permanent. The primary symptom will be loss of motion in the a ected joint(s), eventually followed by unrelenting contraction of the muscles. Depending on the a ected extremity the arm may draw inwards, the leg will curl back into a fetal-like position, or the hand will develop a claw-like appearance. Once well-established the limb cannot be straightened even by the care provider.

Predisposing conditions include burns, trauma, immobility, and deformity. Age itself plays only a very small role. Anyone who is bedfast and who does not possess voluntary movement of their limbs can develop this condition if their muscles and joints are not exercised by stretching and bending.

Prevention is the key to avoiding this condition. You will need to implement a program of early movement and physical therapy in cases of acute or orthopedic injury. Each joint should be exercised separately. In the case of the leg, for instance, the toes, the ankle, the knee, and the hip should all be addressed individually.

Q's and A's:

Thermometers

Q: How do I use a mercury thermometer?

A: Grasp it by the head and shake it in a downward, flinging motion to cause the mercury to settle towards the bulb end. You want it at about 92-94 F – approx. 33 degrees Celsius – before using. The bulb end is then tucked into one of the pockets under either side of the centre of the tongue and held there with lips closed for 8 minutes in order to obtain an accurate reading. This is considered to be an accurate core temp, or equal to the actual temperature inside the body itself. Avoid taking the temp immediately after drinking. A normal temperature is 98.6 F.

Q: What about rectal thermometers?

A: They should be shaken down to the same level and then inserted very gently (use water-soluble lubricant or petroleum jelly, and ideally a plastic sheath) into the rectum. 1 inch is sufficient for infants, 2 inches for adults. Accurate temps are

Contents

obtained after 5 minutes. Rectal temps are generally considered to be 1 degree F warmer than the true core temperature so subtract 1 degree from your reading. Avoid taking the temp immediately after activity, a bowel movement or a bath or shower.

Q: Can I take the temp under the arm?

A: Yes, using an oral thermometer. Prepare it the same way by shaking it down then placing in the pocket of the armpit with the arm held down to the side. Obtaining an accurate axillary temp takes 11 minutes. Axillary temps are considered to be 1 degree F cooler than a true core temp so add 1 degree.

Q: Which site is best?

A: The mouth gives the most accurate core temp reading, and also reacts faster to rising temps than either the rectal or axillary sites.

Q: What is considered a normal healthy body temperature?

A: 98.6 F (37 C) is generally considered to be ideal, with 98.0 to 99.0 the generally accepted "normal" ranges for healthy persons. In the elderly 2 degrees below "normal" that may be their actual normal body temperature. Thus 98.6 may actually represent a fever in some people in these individuals. The key is in knowing what is normal for that person.

Q: What about abnormal temps?

A: 105 F is very high in an adult, potentially life-threatening. In that range damage to the brain, blood, muscles, and kidneys is increasingly likely. Anything over 100 degrees should be addressed. Small children may spike temps of 105 and even 106 for short periods and not suffer ill effects, but as we age our tolerance for fever decreases. 103 is very high in the elderly and cause for serious concern whereas for most adults and even children 104 (40 C) is still relatively safe but bears close watching. In any event active cooling measures should be undertaken before it reaches that level if possible.

Fever

Q: How do I reduce a fever when I don't have medications available?

A: Think in terms of the body's natural cooling mechanisms and make use of them. The human body cools itself by evaporation (sweating), radiation (giving off heat from the body surface) and conduction (transferring heat from a warmer to a cooler surface).

The first thing that can be done is to reduce the coverings over the body, such as clothing and bed linens. This allows for cooling via radiation. Expose as much of the patient's body surface as practical to open air.

Contents

The two most commonly used non-pharmaceutical mechanisms used to reduce fever can be classified as wet and dry treatments.

Wet treatments include sponge baths, cool compresses, and alcohol rubs. By wetting the body surface they increase evaporative heat loss. These work best when the humidity level is 90% or below.

Dry treatments include ice bags and chemical cold packs. The body itself is not made wet; instead cooling is effected by conduction.

A wet method of cooling via conduction is to partially immerse the body no deeper than mid-chest in tepid water (approximately 80 F). Cold water may cause the body

lose too much heat, causing the opposite of fever, or hypothermia. If the water causes shivering the temperature may actually rise instead.

Giving Medications

Q: Why are injections better than tablets?

A: The short answer is they not always are. There are potential complications in administering and using them. Where possible try and avoid using them. However injections are useful when your patient cannot swallow or is nil by mouth (NPO) or you want the medication to work quicker and achieve higher blood levels (i.e. antibiotics in serious infections) or the medicine is broken down in the stomach or not properly absorbed (e.g. adrenaline, insulin). For 95% of patients tablets are fine.

Q: Can I crush tablets and dissolve them in water or put them in jam?

A: Most of the time. The only tablets, which shouldn't be cut up or crushed, are slow release tablets (SR or CR) – these are designed to release the drug slowly over a period of time and part of that mechanism is destroyed if the tablet is crushed or broken.

Q: What can I do for someone who has trouble swallowing pills or capsules that shouldn't be crushed or broken?

A: Placing them in a bit of jam or crushed fruit such as apple, pear or guava (avoid citrus fruits as the acid content may interfere with the medication) and administering them by spoon seems to work for most people.

Q: How do I administer injections?

Contents

Information on giving injections can be found in any basic medical or nursing book. This is simply an overview. There are 3 common sorts of injections.

Subcutaneous – into the subcutaneous layer under the skin using a small short needle (24g). This is very easy to do and the medication is reasonably rapidly absorbed. This route should be avoided in patients who are shocked and with

medications which are strongly chemically irritant e.g. most antibiotics, thiopentone.

- Intramuscular – into a large muscle using a longer slightly larger needle (22 or 20g). The best location for the inexperienced in into the large muscle bulk of the outer aspect of the thigh. Intramuscular injections are reasonably rapidly absorbed, but provide a degree of sustained release effect. Muscle can tolerate more irritant medications (e.g. most antibiotics) but some drugs can cause significant muscle damage if given by IM infection e.g. thiopentone
- Intravenous – into a vein. This is the most rapid route of administration and gives the greatest clinical effect. It is much easier to slowly adjust the dose of a medication using the route, but the effects of giving too much of a drug are much more pronounced.

There is a danger of allergic reaction anytime a medication is given – but it is most pronounced with IV administration. Anytime you administer a medication you should be prepared to treat an allergic reaction. Most are simply a red itchy rash or facial swelling. Usually they are self-limiting. Occasionally the reaction is more severe and evolves to an anaphylactic reaction – involving abdominal pain, vomiting, difficulty breathing, low blood pressure, or swelling in the throat. This is life threatening and is treated with an IM injection of adrenaline. Management of this is well covered in the main references.

Measuring the Pulse

Q: How do I check the pulse?

A: The pulse can be checked at the vertical notch of the neck next to the throat (carotid artery), the inside wrist (radial artery), in the groin, behind the knee, and on the top of the foot. As a general rule of thumb the weaker the blood pressure the higher you'll have to check for a pulse, though there is no concrete rule indicating what level of blood pressure will result in a pulse at what site. A pulse can also be heard using a stethoscope placed over the left chest above the heart (called an apical pulse). Either count for a full minute or for 30 seconds and multiply x2 to determine the pulse rate. Pulses are always expressed in beats per minute.

Contents

Q: What is a normal pulse rate?

A: This varies widely amongst any population, depending upon the presence of pre- existing disease, physical conditioning, whether the person was at rest prior to assessing the rate or recently active, and more. As a general rule pulses between 60 and 100 are considered normal for most adults. Normal rates are best determined in the absence of pain, illness, and injury, while the person is at rest. Absent that you will need to measure the pulse rate over a period of time to arrive at a likely norm with significant variances from that indicating potential problems.

Weight

Q: What does short-term weight loss or gain indicate?

A: This may mean a gradual change in fluid retention or loss, or poor nutritional status. Look for additional clues such as fluid intake exceeding output by more than 20%, or loss via urination exceeding intake by the same amount. Likewise match weight loss or gain over a period of weeks to nutritional intake. Ideally weight fluctuations should not exceed +/- 1 pound (0.5 Kilos) per day in an otherwise healthy individual whose fluid and nutritional intakes are in balance with body requirements.

Q: How do I measure the weight of someone who is unable to stand unassisted?

A: Perhaps the simplest method is to use a chair. Place a platform on the scale to hold the chair, then the empty chair itself. Weight this and write it down. Now place the patient in the chair and weigh them. By subtracting the weight of the empty chair, etc. from the total you have the weight of the patient. Make sure you use the same chair, etc. each time, or your results will be in error.

Elimination Needs

Q: What are the basic tools needed to address bodily elimination needs?

A: The primary tools are the bedpan, the urinal, the rectangular basin, and the hot water bottle. Virtually all elimination needs can be addressed with these items and a few accessories such as soap and washcloths. Bedpans come in two basic forms; the wedge-shaped fracture pan and the traditional deep bedpan. Urinals are used mostly for male patients; though specially designed female urinals are available they are rarely seen. The rectangular basin serves as a multi-use container for washing and emesis catchment. It is far less prone to spilling than kidney-shaped emesis basins and also eliminates one extra item from your inventory. Hot water bottles serve well as reusable enema bags as well as other uses not specifically related to elimination.

Q: Which is better, a fracture pan or a regular bedpan?

Contents

A: Fracture pans are usually the most convenient for women and children but they are limited in capacity and tend to spill more easily when removed. A traditional deep bedpan is more comfortable when fractures to the hips, pelvis or upper leg or back pain are not involved. In such cases a fracture pan, which is wedge shaped, is more comfortable for the patient. Males will find either style usable with the previous caveats in mind.

Q: What about someone who can stand but isn't able to walk to the toilet?

A: A bedside commode can be fashioned from a sturdy chair that has had an oval or round hole cut in the seat and a basin affixed underneath that can be easily removed for emptying. When properly placed at the bedside the patient can stand, or be stood with assistance, pivoted and sat upon the chair. Arms on the chair will make

movement easier for someone who has the ability to support himself or herself using their upper body but may interfere with their ability to transfer onto the chair.

Q: How about urinals?

A: Urinals are used most often by male patients for passing urine. They can be readily improvised from a coffee can or jar though the manufactured version is designed with an angle to the neck so that urine does not spill when the device is used. For male patients and caregivers alike they are easier to use than a bedpan. Female urinals are rarely used but are available. The bedpan is normally used for women.

Q: What is the best way to handle vomiting?

A: While so-called emesis basins (kidney-shaped plastic or metal pans) are available they are of limited capacity and spill readily. Better suited is a basin of approximately 6 inches depth and rectangular in shape. It holds more and doesn't tend to allow a forceful vomit to splash out of the container.

Another alternative is a plastic bag such as a small dustbin or wastebasket liner. A 6 or 8-inch diameter embroidery hoop will hold it open and give the patient something to hang on to. To close it merely grasp the bag with one hand and twist the hoop around with the other. Once removed from the hoop frame it can be sealed using string or a metal twist-tie. The plastic bag has the advantage of being flexible and semi-spill proof, as well as easily disposed of.

Another expedient holder is a wire coat hanger pulled open to form a diamond shape to which the plastic liner has been securely taped.

Q: What about underpads?

Contents

A: Underpads or incontinence pads are reusable mats made of absorbent material – usually cotton with a moisture-proof backing – that are placed underneath the patient to catch and absorb urine. They also prevent faeces from contaminating bed linens and make cleanup easier. Also consider using a plastic or rubber under mat to protect the mattress.

Q: Aren't there disposable ones too?

A: Yes, often referred to by the now generic term "chux." They are intended for one- time use then disposed of. While they work well within their limits perspiration alone can render them ready for disposal, causing the expenditure of large quantities in a very short period of time.

Q: Can you explain what you mean about hot water bottles?

A: Sometimes referred to as an enema syringe or a douche bag, simply described it is a latex rubber or plastic bottle with a stopper that either seals it completely or allows attachment of a hose, which in turn is fitted to one of an assortment of tips designed for differing purposes. Used to administer an enema, for instance, one would fill it with the solution of choice such as warm water and soap suds, introduce the proper tip

into the rectum, and allow the contents of the bag to flow into the rectum by gravity feed.

Q: What about cleaning up afterwards?

A: Soap and water combined with a washing cloth work best. A gentle, non-irritating soap without added antibacterial agents is all that is needed. You may also wish to consider using pre-moistened cloths (also known as baby wipes, etc). These are simply pre-wetted disposable cloths used to clean faeces, urine, and emesis. Large sizes are available for health care use but the smaller version made for cleaning up babies will also suffice. Good quality paper towels can used to fashion wipes by adding soap and water to a basin, tossing in the paper towels to absorb the mixture, and then wringing out the excess water and placing them in plastic bags for later use. Do not overlook toilet tissue as the most basic aid to cleaning up.

Remember urine, faeces, and emesis are all potential disease carriers. Therefore, gloves for the caregiver are a must. You will use more gloves for purposes of cleaning up patients requiring hygiene assistance than you are ever likely to use for addressing wounds or performing other procedures. The bedpans, urinals and basins themselves should be cleaned with soap and water after use and set out to dry or they will be come a source of unwelcome odours.

Pacing Yourself

You will do your patient no good if you work to the point of exhaustion. Learn to sleep when your patient sleeps. Have someone else watch over the patient while you sleep if you can't arrange to sleep when your patient does. The helper can notify you of any emergency or other need such as pain medication.

Establish a routine. If the patient's condition is acute but not urgent and regular vital signs are called for set a schedule. A generally accepted standard is every 4 – 8 hours. For more serious cases whose condition may change regularly use the shorter interval, such as trauma cases or very acute illness. For a patient who is recovering usually every 8 hours is frequent enough unless there is an unexpected change, at which time you may want to reassess the current vital signs.

Look for shortcuts. Instead of placing the patient in bed fully clothed provide them with a modest cover. This facilitates faster access for dressing changes and elimination needs and also reduces the laundry load. Try arranging the schedule of cares so that you can accomplish several tasks in one visit to the bedside. If caring for several patients at once schedule their cares in blocks of time that allow progression from one individual to another once the bulk of the needed treatments have been completed.

Place a hand bell or other audible signaling device where the person can reach if it they need something. Arrange a pull cord so that a bell will ring when assistance is required. This will allow you to tend to other patients or even to spend much-needed time away from the sickroom without the patient lacking for attention when required.

Have a family member or friend sit with them and provide simple services such as adjusting bedding and pillows, or feeding them or assisting with simple tasks that do not require a trained caregiver.

Focus on effect and outcomes instead of perfect technique. For persons formally trained in nursing technique this may represent a major mental obstacle to overcome. Lack of the tools and on-call resources that are routinely at our disposal in a modern, working healthcare system can be frustrating at best, and disabling if we dwell upon what we do not have versus what is available.

In providing nursing care in the austere environment we need to focus on the patient first and foremost. There should be no artificial schedules such as demanded by an institution. Your actions should be focused on the one or few patients under your care.

The one overriding consideration that needs to be reinforced is this: model your care around that necessary for the comfort and recovery of your patient(s) and not around any medical-legal model of what care should be for a given case. Base your actions on what is in the patient's best interests at all times. Do no harm, know what is harmful, and proceed accordingly.

Chapter 17 Frequently asked questions

There are a number of recurring questions, which appear when people are discussing preparedness medicine in various discussion forums which haven't been covered elsewhere in this book. Here we have tried to provide a brief answer to some of the common question coupled with more detailed references for those who are interested.

- 1. What is Ketamine?

Contents

Ketamine is a general anaesthetic agent with unique properties. It has gained a reputation as street drug and as a Vet anaesthetic, but is also widely used in human medicine, and is an ideal anaesthetic agent for austere situations.

It produces a state known as "dissociative anaesthesia" – meaning it produces conditions suitable for performing painful procedures and operations while the patient appears to be in a semi-awake state although unresponsive. A side effect of this anaesthetic state is relative preservation of airway reflexes, respiratory effort, and a stable cardiovascular profile.

It can be administered by intramuscular or intravenous injection or intravenous infusion. It is contraindicated in patients with an allergy to it (rare), and should be used with care in patients with psychiatric history, and patients with severe head injuries. Its main side effect is "emergence agitation" as the patient is waking up from the anaesthetic they may hallucinate and become agitated – this can be minimised by waking the patient up in quite dark environment, and can be treated with benzodiazepines (Valium).

It also causes an increase in respiratory secretions and can cause transient increase in muscle tone.

Due to its ease of use and lack of airway or respiratory suppression it is the ideal drug for use in an austere environment. It has been used extensively in the third world and has an excellent safety profile in comparison to other anaesthetic agent.

In some States in the US, Ketamine is specially controlled because of its use as an illicit "date rape" drug. Unlawful possession of it is a serious felony.

Reference. www.emedicine.com/emerg/topic802.htm

- ### 1. How do I debride a wound?

This is an extract from the US Special Forces Medical Handbook published in 1982 – it contains a chapter on War surgery, which covers debridement of wounds well, and

aspects of wounds to other organ systems – and unfortunately was not included in the new edition:

" 16.2 Soft Tissue Injuries

Contents

1. *In the following surgical procedures we will assume that the medic knows how to prepare a patient for surgery and set up a surgical field*
2. *The primary objective in the treatment of soft tissue injuries is localisation or isolation of deleterious effects of the injury. To best accomplish this objective, remove all foreign substances and devitalised tissues and maintain an adequate blood supply to the injured part. This can be achieved by a 2 step procedure:*
   1. *Step one is a through debridement of the injured area, accomplished as soon as possible after the injury (when delay is unavoidable, systemic antibiotics should be started) The wound should be left open (with a few exceptions) to granulate.*
   2. *Step two is a delayed primary closure within 4-10 days after injury. The wound must be kept clean during this time and antibiotics are usually indicated. The indication for delayed primary closure is the clean appearance of the wound during this time.*
3. *Antibiotic wound therapy. This should be started prior to debridement.*
   1. *Penicillin – 10 million units IV q8hrs for 3 days*
   2. *Kanamycin – 500mg IM q12hrs for 3 days – then review*

<< Editors note. Current military recommendations for antibiotic therapy for wounds is Cefotetan 2gm given every 12 hours >>

- 1. *Tetanus Toxoid 0.5 ml IM once*

1. *Debridement*
   1. *An incision is made in the skin and fascia long enough to give good exposure. Good exposure is required to allow adequate evaluation. Incisions should be made over the wound (both entrance and exit wounds in GSW's) along the longitudinal axis of extremities (s-shaped if crossing joints). Avoid making and incision over superficial bones. When excising skin only, cut 2-3 cm from the wound edge.*
   2. *Skin, fascia, and muscle should be separated to give adequate exposure. Muscles should be separated into there groups and each muscle group debrided separately.*
   3. *Distinguishing tissue viability. Use the 4 C's – Colour, Consistency, Contractility and circulation. With colour being the least desirable*

Contents

	Viable	*Dead or Dying*
Colour	Bright reddish brown	Dark, Cyanotic
Consistency	Springy	Mushy
Contractility	Contracts when cut or pinched	Does not contract
Circulation	Bleeds when cut	Does not bleed

Contents

- *Steps of Debridement. All devitalised muscle must be removed; if not the chance of infection is greater. It is better to take good muscle and have some deformity, than to leave devitalised muscle and have infection. The preferred method for debridement is to cut along one side of a muscle group in strips or blocks and not piecemeal*

    1. *Remove all blood clots, foreign material, and debris from the wound during exploration of the wound with a gloved finger.*
    2. *Vital structures like major blood vessels and nerves must be protected from damage.*
    3. *All procedures must be carried out gently with precision and skill*
    4. *Major blood vessels must be repaired promptly*
    5. *All foreign bodies must be removed, including small detached bone fragments, but time must no be wasted looking for elusive metallic fragments which would require more extensive dissection.*
    6. *Tendons usually do not require extensive debridement. Trim loose frayed edges and ends. Repair should not be performed during initial treatment.*
    7. *Haemostasis must be precise*
    8. *Repeated irrigation of the wound with physiological salt solution <or water if no alternative – although this isn't ideal> during the operation will keep the wound clean and free of foreign material. THIS STEP CANNOT BE OVER EMPHASIZED*
    9. *When debridement is complete, all blood vessels, nerves, and tendons should be covered with soft tissue to protect from drying out.*
    10. *Joint synovium should be closed or at least the joint capsule. The skin and SC tissues is left open in any case*
    11. *Dependent drainage of deep wounds must be employed << Place a Penrose drain (rubber tube) or wicking gauze into the wound>>.*
    12. *Liberal fasciotomy of an extremity is often an additional precaution that allows for post operative swelling. Use when the 5 P are present distal to a limb injury – pain, pallor, pulselessness, puffiness or paraesthesia*
    13. *Do not dress the wound with an occlusive dressing, but place a few strips of fine-mesh gauze between the walls of the wound, placed puffed gauze in the pocket formed and then dress the wound to protect, but not constrict.*
    14. *All wounds should be left open with the exception of wounds of the face, sucking chest wounds, head wounds of the joints or synovial membranes, and*